Orthopedic Examination

A Step by Step Guide

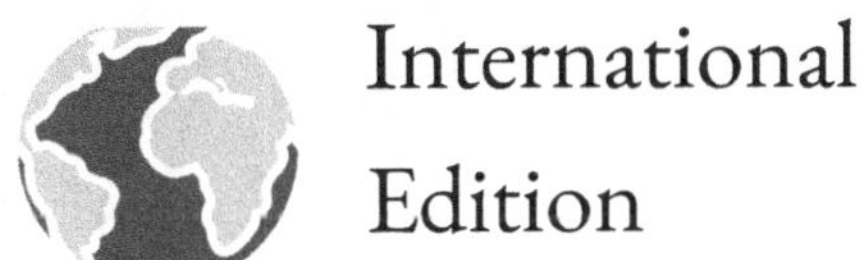

International Edition

Published by Epomedicine

Dr. Sulabh Kumar Shrestha

Dr. Sulabh Kumar Shrestha

Consultant Orthopedic Surgeon
MS Orthopedics & Trauma

Dr. Sulabh Kumar Shrestha is a Nepali orthopedic surgeon and medical educator who is known for creating concise and easy-to-understand notes on various medical topics which are popular among medical students and professionals. Some of the resources he has shared online include:

1. Epomedicine.com
   - A website with topics & mnemonics dedicated to medical students and professionals

2. Neuroanatomy notes (2021)
   - Neuroanatomy simplified with diagrams & mnemonics

3. Uncolored Thoughts (2023)
   - A poetry collection

Email: res.sulabhkumarshrestha@pahs.edu.np

Website: sulabhkshrestha.com.np

Orthopedic Examination - A Step by Step Guide (International Edition)

© 2024 by Dr. Sulabh Kumar Shrestha

Published by Epomedicine

All rights reserved.

This book contains images that are in the public domain as well as images licensed under the Creative Commons Attribution 4.0 International License (CC BY 4.0). For the CC BY 4.0 images, proper attribution has been provided as per the license requirements.

Disclaimer: The author and the publisher have made every effort to ensure that the information in this book is correct and complete. The advice and strategies contained herein may not be suitable for every situation. Neither the author nor the publisher shall be liable for any loss of profit or any other commercial damages, including but not limited to special, incidental, consequential, or other damages.

For any permissions or inquiries, please contact:

Epomedicine

webmaster@epomedicine.com

Reference books & Further reading:

1. Orthopaedic Examination Techniques : A practical guide (3rd edition)
Fazal Ali, Nick Harris - 2022

2. Clinical Orthopaedic Examination (6th edition)
Ronal McRae - 2010

3. Handbook of Clinical Examination in Orthopedics : An illustrated guide
Sarvdeep S. Dhatt, Sharad Pravakar - 2019

4. Practical Orthopedic Examination Made Easy (2nd edition)
Manish Kumar Varshney - 2012

5. Apley & Solomon's System of Orthopedics and Trauma (10th edition)
Ashley Blom, David Warwick, Michael Whitewhouse - 2017

6. Miller's Review of Orthopedics (8th edition)
Mark D. Miller, Stephen R. Thompson - 2019

7. The Knee Made Easy
Charlambos Panayiotou Charlambous - 2021

8. The Shoulder Made Easy
Charlambos Panayiotou Charlambous - 2019

9. Clinical Examination in Orthopedic
K Mohan Iyer - 2012

Preface

Whether you are an orthopedic surgeon, physical therapist, or medical student, this book serves as an invaluable resource for enhancing your clinical practice.

This book has four sections: Section 1 details the principles of history taking and general examination in orthopedic patients; Section 2 covers examination of the joints and the spine; Section 3 deals with examination of the peripheral nerves of the hand; Section 4 discusses making differential diagnoses.

The chapters are organized in a logical and easy-to-follow manner, with numerous illustrations and photographs to aid readers in understanding the material.

This book comprises content in bullets and mnemonics which is expected to be easier to understand, follow and recall during patient assessment.

S.K.S

Epomedicine

2024

Table of Contents

Section 3 : Peripheral nerves

Section 4 : DxD

Abbreviations

1. **ACJ: Acromioclavicular joint**
2. **ACL: Anterior Cruciate Ligament**
3. **ADM: Abductor Digiti Minimmi**
4. **AIN: Anterior Interosseous Nerve**
5. **ALL: Anterolateral Ligament**
6. **ALRI: Anterolateral Rotatory Instability**
7. **AMRI: Anteromedial Rotatory Instability**
8. **APB: Abductor Pollicis Brevis**
9. **APL: Abductor Pollicis Longus**
10. **AS: Ankylosing Spondylitis**
11. **ASIS: Anterior Superior Iliac Spine**
12. **ATFL: Anterior Talofibular Ligament**
13. **BCC: Basal Cell Carcinoma**
14. **BR: Brachioradialis**
15. **CAGE: Cut, Annoyed, Guilty & Eye**
16. **CFL: Calcaneofibular Ligament**
17. **CMCJ: Carpometacarpal Joint**
18. **CRT: Capillary refill time**
19. **DIPJ: Distal interphalangeal joint**
20. **DTR: Deep Tendon Reflex**
21. **ECRB: Extensor Carpi Radialis Brevis**
22. **ECRL: Extensor Carpi Radialis Longus**

23. **ECU: Extensor Carpi Ulnaris**

24. **EDC: Extensor Digitorum Communis**

25. **EDM: Extensor Digitroum Minimmi**

26. **EHL: Extensor Hallucis Longus**

27. **EIP: Extensor Indicis Proprius**

28. **EPB: Extensor Pollicis Brevis**

29. **EPL: Extensor Pollicis Longus**

30. **FAI: Femoroacetabular Impingement**

31. **FCR: Flexor Carpi Radialis**

32. **FCU: Flexor Carpi Ulnaris**

33. **FDP: Flexor Digitorum Profundus**

34. **FDS: Flexor Digitorum Superficialis**

35. **FPA: Foot Progression Angle**

36. **FPL: Flexor Pollicis Longus**

37. **GCT: Giant Cell Tumor**

38. **GT: Greater trochanter/tuberosity**

39. **ITB: Iliotibial band**

40. **LCL: Lateral Collateral Ligament**

41. **LLD: Limb Length Discrepancy**

42. **MCL: Medial Collateral Ligament**

43. **MCPJ: Metacarpophalangeal joint**

44. **MRC: Medical Research Council**

45. **MTPJ: Metatarsophalangeal Joint**

46. **OCD: Osteochondritis Dissecans**

47. **OP: Opponens Pollicis**

48. **ORL: Oblique Retinacular Ligament**

49. **PCL: Posterior Cruciate Ligament**

50. **PIN: Posterior Interosseous Nerve**

51. **PIPJ: Proximal interphalangeal joint**

52. **PL: Palmaris Longus**

53. **PLC: Posterolateral Corner**

54. **PLRI: Posterolateral Rotatory Instability**

55. **PMRI: Posteromedial Rotatory Instability**

56. **PSIS: Posterior Superior Iliac Spine**

57. **PTFL: Posterior Talofibular Ligament**

58. **Q-angle: Quadriceps angle**

59. **ROM: Range of Motion**

60. **RTS: Radial Tunnel Syndrome**

61. **SCC: Squamous Cell Carcinoma**

62. **SIJ: Sacroiliac joint**

63. **SL: Scapholunate**

64. **SLRT: Straight Leg Raising Test**

65. **TB: Tuberculosis**

66. **TFCC: Triangular Fibrocartilage Complex**

67. **VMO: Vastus Medialis Obliquus**

68. **VPMRI: Varus Posteromedial Rotatory Instability**

CHAPTER 1

History taking in Orthopedics

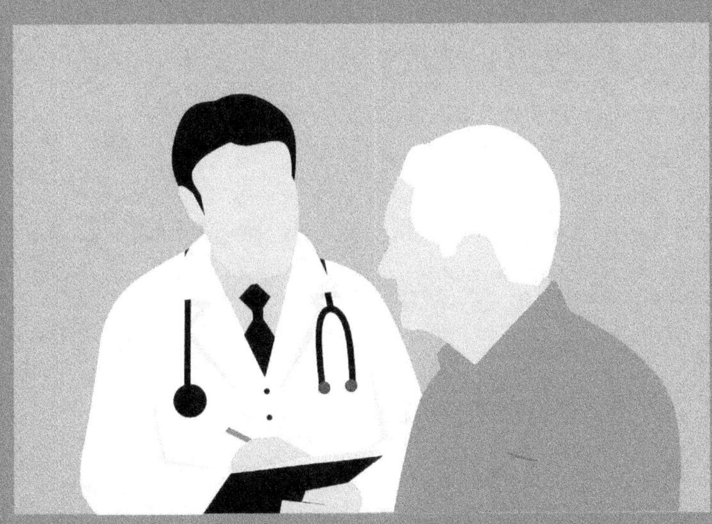

History taking in Orthopedics

Orthopedic history taking is a crucial step in the evaluation of patients with musculoskeletal disorders or injuries. A thorough and systematic approach to taking a patient's history can help identify the underlying cause of the problem, guide further evaluation, and inform treatment decisions.

General approach to history taking with patients has been discussed here:

https://epomedicine.com/clinical-medicine/history-taking-sequence-and-mnemonics/

So, a general strategy in an orthopedic history taking includes eliciting the following:

Chief complaint

Common orthopedic complaints can be remembered using the mnemonic **WRISD Pain** –

- <u>Weakness:</u> May be due to –

    - Pain inhibition

    - Muscle strain

    - Neurologic interruption

- <u>Restricted movement (stiffness):</u> May be due to –

    - Pain and muscle spasm (Pseudo-locking)

    - Stretching of soft tissue contracture

    - Mechanical blockage by osteophytes, loose bodies or bucket-handle meniscal tears (Locking)

- <u>Redness (Erythema) or warmth:</u> May be due to –

    - Trauma

    - Acute infection

    - Acute inflammatory process (e.g. Gout)

- <u>Instability (giving away or jumping out of place):</u> May be due to –

    - Traumatic damage of muscular, capsular or ligamentous structures

    - Inherent laxity

    - More apparent when the joint is positioned such that muscles have less mechanical advantage (overhead shoulder positions) or when a quick movement demand is faster than the reaction time for corresponding muscles (cutting or rotatory knee movements)

- <u>Swelling:</u> May be –
  - Traumatic and rapid appearance: Hematoma or Hemarthrosis
  - Slow appearance: Inflammation, Joint effusion, Infection, Tumor
  - Painful: Active inflammation, Infection, Tumor
- <u>Sensory disturbance (numbness or paresthesia):</u> May be due to –
  - Pressure from neighboring structure into nerve (e.g. PIVD)
  - Local ischemia of nerve (nerve entrapment)
  - Peripheral neuropathy
- <u>Deformity:</u> May be related to –
  - Shortening
  - Lengthening
  - Malalignment

- Swelling (e.g. effusion or intramuscular hematoma)
- <u>Disability (functional loss)</u>
- <u>Pain:</u> May be –
    - Local pain (bone pain is deep pain commonly worse in evening)
    - Referred pain:
        - From scleratogenous sources (nondermatomal pattern with no hard neurologic findings): e.g. facet and disc generated pain
        - From visceral sources (will have visceral complaints) e.g. cholelithiasis, cardiac ischemia
    - Autonomic pain: vague, widespread and often associated with vasomotor and trophic changes

History of presenting illness

Remember the mnemonic **"SOCRATES"** which was classically used for pain assessment.

Headings	Questions
Site	Where is the [symptom]?
Onset	1. **Acute or Gradual or Acute on chronic?** 2. **Traumatic or Atraumatic?** – If traumatic: a. Fall? (fracture/dislocation/contusion) b. Excessive stress? (ligament/capsule or muscle/tendon pathology) c. Sudden axial traction to joint? (subluxation/dislocation) d. Axial compression to joint? (fracture/synovitis) e. Twisting? (meniscal injury) f. Associated sound? (snap/tear/pop/clicking/clunk) g. Associated swelling? (immediate/after short interval) h. Ability to mobilize in immediate post-injury time? 3. **History of overuse?** a. Position in which he/she works? b. Repetitive work or sports movements?

Character	How would you describe the [symptom]? 1. **Pain:** Dull/Sharp/Burning? 2. **Locking:** Catching/Jamming/Noise? At movement/rest? Position of locking? Sudden/gradual unlocking? 3. **Instability:** Sudden loss of control/wobbly/buckles/shifts? On standing/movement? Fallen down/short of falling down? 4. **Stiffness:** Global/specific movement? 5. **Weakness:** Global/specific movement? Global/specific limb position? Affecting high/low demand activities? 6. **Sensory disturbance:** Altered sensation/pins-needles/reduced sensation/tingling/numbness/'dead' arm or leg? 7. **Swelling**
Radiation	Does the [symptom] spread elsewhere? Is the [symptom] present at other sites?

Associated symptoms	1. **Other symptoms:** Pain, Instability, Weakness, Swelling, Deformity, Limping, Sensory disturbance, etc. – may be isolated or present in combination 2. **Impact:** Helps to gauze limitation of patient and level of intervention necessary – a. Functional limitations: Activities of daily living? Occupational limitations? Recreational limitations? b. Effect on personal and social life? c. Effect on psychological well being? 3. **Red flags:** Presence indicates the pathology is not benign & suggests underlying pathology – a. Unexplained weight loss (>10 pounds in 3 months) or loss of appetite b. Previous history of cancer c. Failure to improve after 1 month of treatment d. Relentless night pain or Pain preventing sleep e. Fever/chills/malaise f. IV drug abuse g. Prolonged steroid use h. Age >50 years i. Significant progressive neurological change or sudden loss of bowel/bladder function
Treatment	What has been tried? (how? by whom? how many times?) What has helped and what has failed?

Timing	1. **Duration:** a. Length? b. Constant/Intermittent? 2. **Change in pattern/size/shape** over time & with joint motion?
Exacerbating & relieving factors	Limb position? Rest/activity? Weight bearing/Non-weight bearing? Walking/running? Walking on a flat surface/ascending or descending stairs? Walking on even/uneven surface? Specific activities (carrying/kneeling/turning/jumping)? Timing (night/day? morning/rest of day?)
Severity	Can be graded in scale of **0 to 10** OR Grade I (mild): Ignorable Grade II (moderate): Interferes with function and needs intermittent attention or treatment Grade III (severe): Invariably present and needs invariable attention or treatment Grade IV (excruciating): Incapacitating

Past History

- Musculoskeletal:
    - Symptomatic joint/limb
    - Opposite joint/limb
    - Other joints

- ■ Inflammatory or other arthropathy
- ■ Previous injuries – fractures or otherwise
- <u>Medical:</u> To identify risk factors of the anesthesia & of surgery morbidity to determine whether the conditions have been brought into the best possible control to minimize the risk.
  - ■ DM (risk of infection)
  - ■ Cardiovascular and respiratory problems (surgical fitness)
  - ■ Malignancy (metastases or recurrence)
  - ■ Infection in other parts of the body
  - ■ Osteonecrosis in other parts of the body
  - ■ DVT/PE (increased postoperative risk)
  - ■ Mouth ulcers, Rashes, Eye symptoms, Urological symptoms (Rheumatoid or Seronegative arthropathies)
- <u>Surgical:</u>
  - ■ Previous surgeries on limb or joint in question
  - ■ Other surgeries
  - ■ Surgical or Anesthetic complications
- <u>Additional for pediatric patients:</u> Ask about problems during –

- Pregnancy (pre-natal history)

- Delivery (birth history)

- Time after delivery (post-natal history)

- Growth history and Developmental milestones

Remember a few key milestones, which will be useful for most consultations.

https://epomedicine.com/medical-students/developmental-milestones-mnemonic/

Age (months)	Milestones
1-2	Holds up chin
6-8	Sits alone
8-10	Stands with support
10-12	Walks with support
14	Walks without support
24	Ascends stairs one foot at a time

Drug History

Remember the mnemonic **"DRUGS"**.

1.   **Doctor prescribed** (including anticoagulants, antiplatelet drugs and fluoroquinolones)
2.   **Recreational** (including anabolic steroids, illicit drugs)
3.   **User** (over the counter purchases, alternative/traditional medicines)
4.   **Gynecological** (contraceptives, HRTs)
5.   **Sensitivities** (exact nature of response and allergies)

Record the medication or drug history in tabulated manner as presented below:

Drugs	Indication	Dose	Preparation	Compliance

Record any walking aids, orthotics and prosthesis used by the patient. Record any known allergies.

Some drugs and their adverse effects affecting the limbs:

DRUG	THERAPEUTIC USE	SIDE EFFECTS
Beta-blockers	Hypertension	Limb coldness
Calcium channel blockers	Hypertension	Ankle edema
ACE Inhibitors	Hypertension	Muscle cramps
Propranolol	Hypertension	Paresthesia
Furosemide	Hypertension	Bullous eruptions
OCPs	Contraception	Risk of DVT
Colchicine	Gout	Neuropathy
Indomethacin	Arthritis	Neuropathy
Corticosteroids	Inflammation	Osteoporosis,
Aspirin	Pain management	Purpura
Metronidazole	Anaerobic infections	Neuropathy
Fluoroquinolones	Infection	Cartilage damage
Vit A & D	Supplement	Ectopic calcification

Family History

1.   **Musculoskeletal:**

     i.   Familial conditions of affected limbs/joints

     ii.   Familial association of osteonecrosis or inflammatory arthropathy (RA, Seronegative arthropathies, Gout)

2.   **Malignancies:** to assess risk of malignancy or bone metastases in patient

	Female	Male	Not specified
Individual	○	□	◇
Affected Individual	●	■	◆
Deceased Individual	⊘	◺	⬦
Carrier (note that carriers are not always marked on a pedigree; often they are simply shown as unaffected)	◐	◧	◈

Symbols used in constructing a pedigree chart by Melissa Hardy, CC BY 4.0

Social History

Mnemonic – "**LOST in Alcohol and Smoking**".

1. Living conditions
2. Occupation
3. Sporting hobbies
4. Travel
5. Alcohol
6. Smoking

1. Alcohol intake and Smoking:

	Alcohol intake	**Smoking**
Assessment method	Units per week "CAGE" questionnaire	Smoke years
Associated orthopedic problems	Non-union (OR 2.5); Deep SSI (OR 2.04); Undefined SSI (OR 3.11)	Delayed union (MD 12·85 weeks); SSI (OR 1.72-2.17)
Other perioperative complication	Cardiopulmonary complications, Bleeding episodes, Alcohol withdrawal	Impaired wound healing, Cardiopulmonary complications
Other risks	Osteonecrosis, Gout	Malignancies

SSI: Surgical Site Infection; OR: Odds Ratio; MD: Mean Difference

2. **Living conditions:**

- Will this patient's home environment be safe for them post-operatively?
- Are there environmental factors contributing to their illness?
- Are there family members at home who can support or care for them?
- Effects of symptoms on daily life (discussed earlier under 'impact' in character of symptom in history of presenting illness)
- Financial

3. **Occupation:**

- Nature of work?
- Is this patient still able to work?
- Any aids/footwear required for the patient during work?

4. **Sports and hobbies:** Details of any sporting hobby should therefore be sought from the patient (to inform about time to avoid sports, time to return to sports and also about necessary warm up exercises)

5. **Travel:**

- Recent travel to tropical countries?

- Foot injuries sustained while walking barefoot?

ICE History (Patient's Perspective)

- **Ideas** – What they think it might be?

- **Concerns** – What they fear it might be?

- **Expectations** – What do they hope or want next to happen?

CHAPTER 2

Equipments in Examination

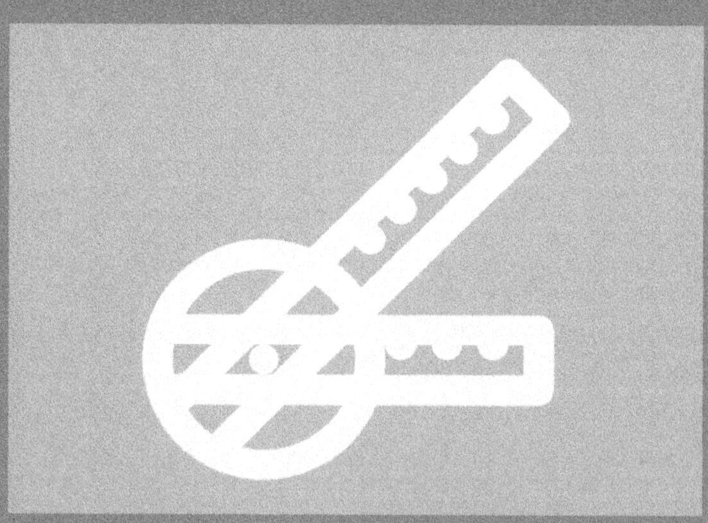

Equipments for examination

Instruments play a crucial role in clinical examination by providing accurate, standardized, & efficient measurements of physical signs.

The list of items required for a orthopedic examination:

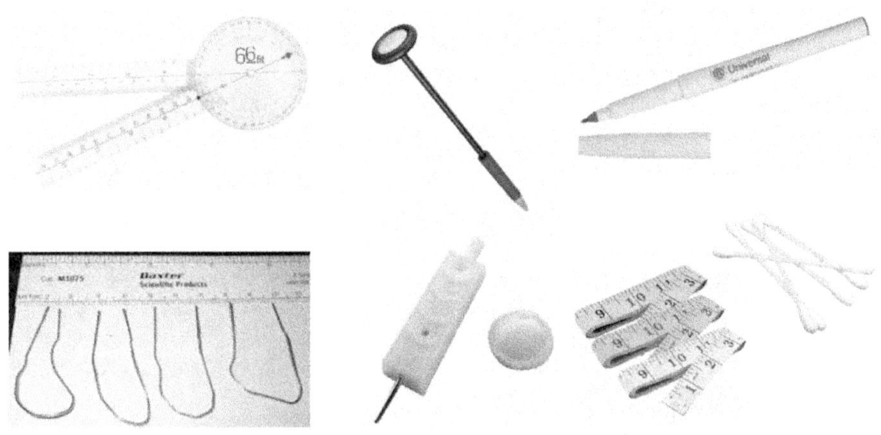

1. **Measuring tape:** For measuring limb length and girth

2. **Goniometer:** For measuring range of motion

- 360 goniometer of different sizes for different joints

- 180 finger goniometer

3. **Tendon hammer:** For eliciting limb reflex and plantar reflex

4. **Skin marking pencil:** For marking important anatomical landmarks

5. **Plumb bob:** To drop a plumb line

6. **128 or 256 Hz tuning fork:** For testing vibration sense and temperature sensation

7. **Disposable sterile sharp points like neurotip:** To assess superficial pain sensation

8. **Cotton wool wisp:** To assess crude or light touch

9. **Paperclip unraveled to create 2 tips set specific distance apart or a compass divider with blunted end:** To test 2-point discrimination

10. **Other general instruments:**

- Stethoscope & Sphygmomanometer
- Pen torch
- Wristwatch
- Clean gloves

CHAPTER 3

Principles of Examination

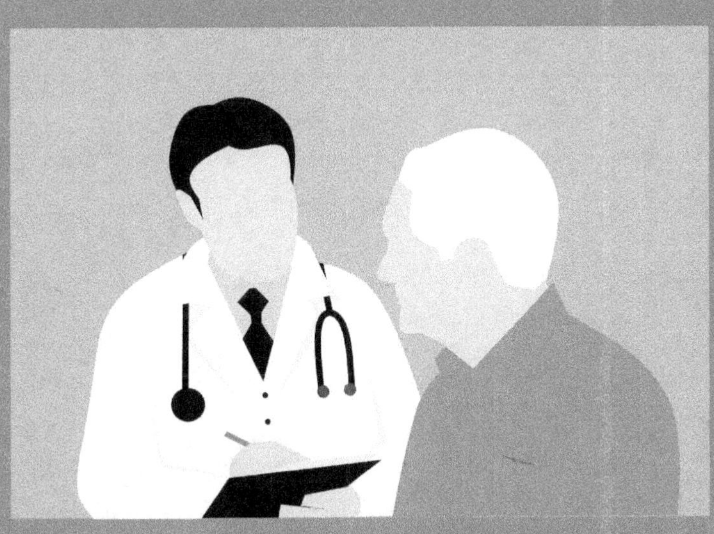

Principles of Examination

The Apley's system of "look, feel, move" or precisely: inspection, palpation, range of motion have been extended to include measurement, neurovascular examination, special tests and completion examination to make the process of examination systematic and complete. All the examinations will be discussed under these headings and will be repeated throughout the book.

Remember **WIPER** before initiating any patient examination.

https://epomedicine.com/clinical-medicine/remember-wiper-before-patient-examination/

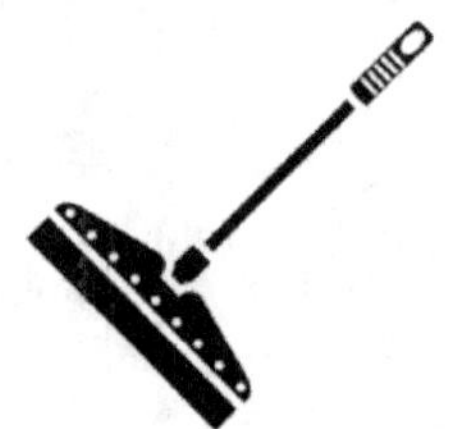

W ash hands (before and after)
I ntroduce yourself to the patient and seek his or her consent
P osition the patient correctly.
E xpose the patient as needed (e.g. 'Please take off your shirt for me now, if that is all right')
R ight side of the bed

The local musculoskeletal examination is carried out following the general physical examination.

The orthopedic examination proceeds in the sequence of: Look, Feel, Move, Measure, Neurovascular examination, Special tests and Neighboring joint examination.

It should flow with patients in: Walking, Standing, Sitting, Supine, Lateral, Prone.

1. Inspection (Look)

Mnemonic: SEADS GO

Look from: Anterior, Sides and Posterior

- **S**kin changes including swelling
- **E**dema
- **A**trophy
- **D**eformity
- **S**hape, **S**ymmetry and **S**hortening
- **G**ait

(https://epomedicine.com/clinical-medicine/physical-examination-gait/)

- **O**rthosis, walking aid, shoes wear

2. Palpation (Feel)

Before palpation, ask the patient to mention the exact site of tenderness as it helps in localizing the site and type of pathology and helps the examiner to remain cautious while palpating the tender area.

Mnemonic: TEST Areas

- **Temperature**
  - Diffuse warmth:
    - Infective or Inflammatory process of joints
    - Anastomotic dilation proximal to an arterial block
  - Localized warmth:
    - Inflammatory process in underlying anatomical structure
  - Asymmetrical coldness:
    - Arterial: Impaired limb circulation
    - Neurological: May also occur during attack of sciatica
- **Effusion**

- **Swelling**

    - Diffuse:

        - Synovial fluid

        - Blood

    - Localized:

        - Soft:

            - Subcutaneous fluid

            - Bursitis

            - Pus

        - Flucuating:

            - Hematoma

            - Mucocele

        - Hardish:

            - Cyst

            - Ganglion

        - Bony:

            - Bony subluxation

            - Callus

            - Osteophyte

            - Bony deformation

- **Tenderness**
  - <u>Greater tenderness when the superficial muscle is tensed:</u> Pathology of superficial muscle
  - <u>Greater tenderness when the superficial muscle is relaxed:</u> Pathology of deeper structures
  - <u>Referred tenderness:</u> Within or near the area of referred pain, it is often possible to find small trigger points which on pressure produces deep and radiating tenderness
    - Cervical dural compression – Upper border of trapezius, scapular muscles or base of neck
    - Lumbar dural compression – Sacroiliac region and upper part of buttocks
  - <u>Associated tenderness:</u> Well-localized tender area very close to the site of the lesion
- **Areas of emphasis**
  - Any deformities
  - Important landmarks

- Joint lines

- Bony points relevant to the joint &
  adjacent ligament/tendon

- Gap: At site of rupture of muscle or tendon

3. Active & Passive Range Of Motion (Move)

- Painful movements at last (to prevent overflow of painful
  movement to next movement)
- Active ROM first, then passive ROM: Following things are
  noted –
  - <u>Range of motion:</u> Angles using goniometer or
    distances between 2 points
    - Stationary arm of goniometer: Lies parallel
      to the stationary segment of limb or
      midline axis of body in some cases
      (shoulder, hip)
    - Mobile arm of goniometer: Placed parallel
      to the axis of the mobile segment of the
      limb

- Center of goniometer: Over central axis of the joint
- <u>Presence of pain:</u> Painful or Painless
    - Pain throughout movement: Acute inflammation or damage to the joint cartilage
    - At the end of the range of movement: Stretching of the capsule, for example, joint effusion.
    - Specific arc of movement: Usually a localized pathology, for example, rotator cuff tears of the shoulder.
- <u>End feel of joint:</u>
    - Physiological:
        - Hard: Movement comes to abrupt stop (bone-to-bone end feel in elbow extension or ligamentous as in knee extension)
        - Elastic (Capsular): Resistance at the end of range but further stretching over few degrees is possible (felt during most rotation movements)

- Tissue approximation: Where extra-articular soft tissue engage with each other (soft muscular feel in elbow or knee flexion)
- Pathological:
    - Too hard (where elastic or tissue approximation is expected): Slight increase in hardness (early arthrosis) to bony block (ankylosing spondylitis)
    - Too soft (where hard is expected): Loose body blocking a movement
    - Muscle spasm: Muscle contraction with sudden vibrant "twang" which occurs due to reflex protective spasm (acute arthritis, recent fracture, etc.)
    - Empty: No organic resistance but stops the movement because of the perceived pain or out of sympathy (acute bursitis, extra-articular abscess, neoplasm, joint laxity or non-organic lesion)

- Springy block: Displaced intra-articular cartilaginous structure preventing full range of motion (displaced meniscus in knee, buckled end-plate in lumbar spine)
  - Crisp: Small involuntary muscle contraction (guarding) at the end of range (cervical disc protrusion)
  - Soggy: Intermediate of soft and empty feeling (rheumatoid arthritis in upper cervical spine)
- Presence of crepitus or clicks:
  - Crepitus (Palpated or Auscultated): Continuous grating sensations produced by movement of rough articular surfaces (osteoarthritis, patellofemoral pain syndrome)
  - Clicks: A tiny, singular noise that occurs during one cycle of movement and it may be produced from –
    - Soft tissues moving over bony prominences (of little importance)

- Soft tissues within the joint (e.g. displaced menisci)

- Disturbances in bony contours (e.g. from intra-articular fractures)

- <u>Movements in abnormal plane:</u> Joint is stressed in a particular plane & excessive movements noted

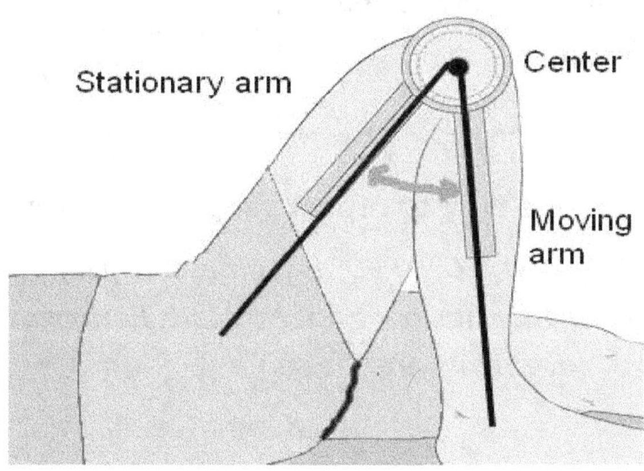

Patterns of limitation in range of motion:

	Intra-articular disease	Periarticular disease
Limitation	Restricted active and passive range of motion	Passive range of motion > Active range of motion (lag sign)
Diseases	Synovitis, Arthritis	Affections of tendons, ligaments, bursa, fascia

	Capsular pattern	Non-capsular pattern
Limitation	Pain & limitation of joint movement in a joint-specific ration	Limitation in a joint in any pattern other than a capsular one
Cause	Arthritis, Prolonged immobilization	Derangement of a part of joint capsule, extra-articular lesion, ligamentous adhesion

Example of a way to report range of motion:

Knee flexion: 0-120°. 0-90° is painless. The remaining 30° is painful. Further flexion is not possible. Both active and passive movements are the same.

	"Fixed" deformity	"Fixed" in deformity
Definition	Arc of movement is limited to 1 direction but full or increased in opposite direction	Limb is fixed in particular degree and direction on neither plane is possible
Example	Fixed flexion deformity of 30° means normal flexion but extension to < 30° is impossible	Fixed in 30° flexion means the limb is in 30° flexion & neither flexion or extension is possible

- **Beighton's score –**

Maneuver	Score
Thumb touches the volar aspect of forearm	1 X 2
Little finger hyperextends parallel to forearm	1 X 2
Elbow hyperextends more than 15°	1 X 2
Knee hyperextends more than 15°	1 X 2
Palm to touch the floor by bending forward with the knee extended	1

≥ 4 of 9 indicates generalized ligament laxity.

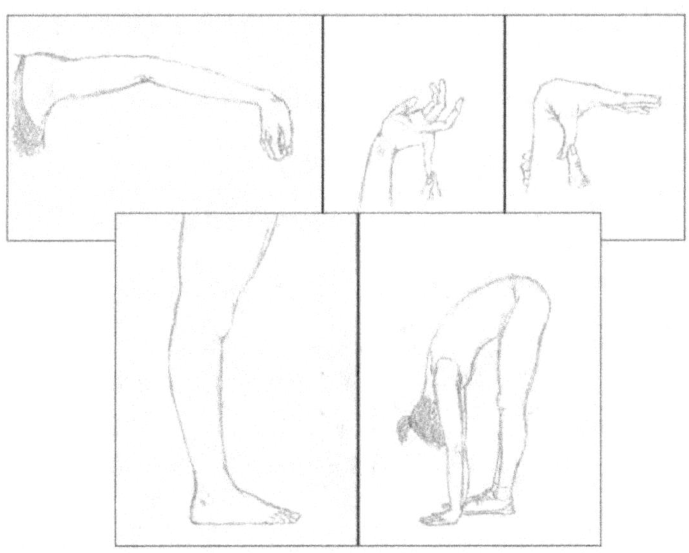

Aleksandra Lacheta, CC BY-SA 4.0, via Wikimedia Commons

4. Measure

- Limb lengths
- Limb circumference
- Specific angles e.g. Carrying angle, Q angle, etc.

4. Neurovascular examination

a. **Motor power and sensations around the joint:**

- <u>Resisted isometric movements:</u> MRC grading –
    - M0 – No contraction
    - M1 – Flickering
    - M2 – Movement with gravity eliminated
    - M3 – Weak movement against gravity
    - M4 – Movement against gravity and partial resistance
    - M5 – Normal power
- <u>Sensation:</u> Light touch, Pin prick, Temperature, Stereognosis, 2 point discrimination, Proprioception; MRC grading –
    - S0 – Absence of all modalities

- S1 – Deep pain sensation
- S2 – Protective skin sensation (skin touch, pain and temperature)
- S3 – S2 with accurate localization
- S3+ – Stereognosis, 2 point discrimination recovery
- S4 – Normal sensation

b. **Peripheral pulsations:** Assess for adequate blood supply

- <u>Dorsalis pedis artery:</u> Just lateral to tendon of EHL (absent in 10%)
- <u>Posterior tibial artery:</u> 2 cm below and posterior to medial malleolus (between FDL and FHL tendons)
- <u>Anterior tibial artery:</u> midway between 2 malleoli against distal tibia, just lateral to EHL tendon
- <u>Popliteal artery:</u> with knee flexed 40 degrees (to relax muscles), in lower part of popliteal fossa against the posterior aspect of tibial condyles
- <u>Femoral artery:</u> just inferior to mid-inguinal point
- <u>Radial artery:</u> at wrist just lateral to FCR tendon
- <u>Brachial artery:</u> just medial to tendon of biceps at elbow

c. **Capillary refill:** Assess for adequate perfusion

- Normal: <2 seconds

d. **Regional lymph nodes:**

- <u>Cervical:</u> submental, submandibular, preauricular, tonsillar, supraclavicular, deep cervical, scalene, posterior auricular, occipital nodes
- <u>Axillary:</u> anterior, central, posterior, lateral and apical groups
- <u>Epitrochlear:</u> medial aspect of elbow, 4-5 cm superior to humeral epitrochlea
- <u>Inguinal:</u>
    - Horizontal chain: just below inguinal ligament
    - Vertical chain: along the line of saphenous vein

5. Special tests

Special tests are unique clinical tests for diagnosis of different pathologies, and these are performed depending on the differential diagnoses in mind.

- **Tests of a particular muscle or musculo-tendinous unit:** Specific position or action to assess power/integrity
- **Provocation tests:** which are designed to be painful in specific conditions
- **Local anesthetic tests:** to remove pain as a cause of dysfunction of a joint or muscle
- **Ligament tests:** to assess stability

6. Examination of adjacent joints

- Always assess the joints above and below the joint or part of examination.
- Any abnormal findings can be reported or if normal – "joints above and below are normal"

Local musculoskeletal examination must be followed by a systemic examination. Thank the patient at the end.

CHAPTER 4

Swelling/Lump Examination

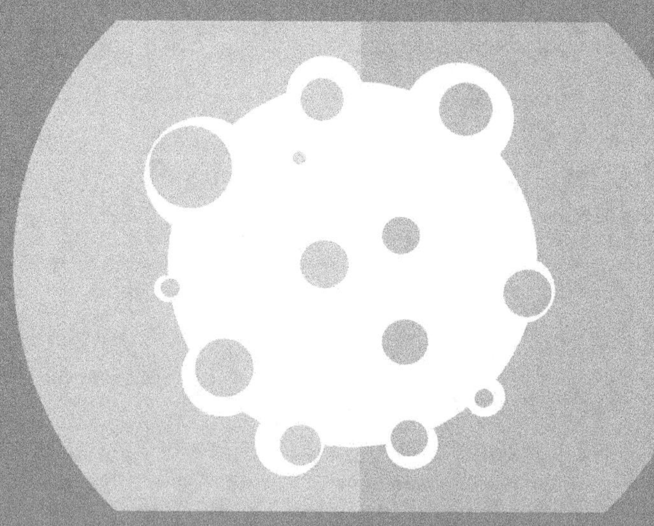

Swelling or Lump Examination

A lump examination is a crucial part of a physical examination where a healthcare provider evaluates the size, shape, texture, and consistency of a lump or swelling to determine its potential cause and significance. A lump can be a benign growth, infection, inflammatory condition or a malignancy.

History (Listen)

Mnemonic: SOCRATES

a. **Site:** Site and Site of origin of lump (in case of huge lumps)

b. **Onset:** Duration (from the time 1st noticed) and Mode (traumatic or spontaneous or from a pre-existing condition like scar)

c. **Constitutional symptoms** (Fever, weight loss, night sweats, etc.) and **Consumption history** (tobacco, betel nut, cigar, etc.)

d. **Recurrence:** Any history of recurrence with or without history of excision

e. **Associated symptoms:** Pain or other systemic complaints (explain further using SOCRATES)

f. **Timing:** Static or Progressive change in size, shape, surface or consistency

g. **Effect:** Activities of Daily Living (ADL), Function (Movements) or Growth plate (Deformity)

h. **Secondary changes:** Softening, Ulceration, Fungation, Inflammatory changes

> **Summary of Lump Examination:**
> 1. History: SOCRATES
> 2. Inspection: 10 S
> 3. Palpation: 6 Students and 3 Teachers around a CAMPFIRE
> 4. Percussion: 3 T
> 5. Auscultation: If pulsatile or peristaltic swelling
> 6. Move, Measure, DNVS
> Tip: Do not forget General Examination

Inspection (Look)

Mnemonic: 10 S

1. Single or multiple

2. Site

3. Size (vertical X horizontal dimensions)

4. Shape (round, oval, irregular)

5. Surface (smooth/irregular, flat/raised)

6. Side/edge (sessile, pedunculated)

7. Shade (color)

8. Skin (redness, ulceration, pigmentation, discharge, punctum, scar, sinus, etc.)

   - Punctum = Sebaceous cyst

9. Surrounding area – distal and proximal (pressure effects: edema, wasting; deformity)

10. Shift (change):

    - <u>Pulsation</u> (Lump arising from artery – expansile pulsation; Lump arising superficial to artery – transmitted pulsation)

- **Peristalsis** (Congenital hypertrophic pyloric stenosis)
- **Impulse with cough** (Swellings in continuity with pleural cavity, abdominal cavity, spinal canal or cranial cavity)
- **Movement with respiration** (Swellings from upper abdominal viscera)
- **Movement with swallowing** (Swellings fixed to larynx or trachea)
- **Movement with protrusion of tongue** (Thyroglossal cyst)

Palpation (Feel)

Mnemonic: 6 Students and 3 Teachers around CAMPFIRE (However, always start examination with and comment on temperature 1st as subsequent palpation can give false rise in temperature.)

1.   **6 S to be stated again:** Site, Size, Shape, Surface, Skin, Shift (including cough or cry impulse)

- Measure the size with measuring tape – vertical and horizontal dimensions
- Mention if portion of swelling disappears behind a bone
- Surface – smooth (cyst), lobular with smooth bumps (lipoma), nodular (matted lymph nodes), irregular/rough (carcinoma)

2. **Temperature (felt with dorsum of fingers):** normal or warm (infection or well-vascularized tumor)

3. **Tenderness** (observe patient's facial expression; lumps from nerves can cause pins and needles)

4. **Transillumination or Translucency:** Darken the room; Roll of X-ray or paper is held on 1 side and observed while the light is held on the other side of the swelling
   - <u>Light is transmitted (Transillumination positive):</u> Lump contains clear fluid (water, serum, lymph, plasma or highly retractile fat)

5. **Consistency:**
   - Uniform
      - <u>Soft (like lips):</u> Lipoma
      - <u>Cystic:</u> Cysts and Chronic abscesses
      - <u>Firm (like nose):</u> Fibroma

- **Hard (like forehead):** Yielding (Chondroma, Dermoid cyst), Bony hard (Osteoma), Stony hard (Carcinoma)
- **Crepitus:** Gaseous swellings (Gas gangrene, surgical emphysema)
- Variable: Malignancy

6.   **Attachment and Mobility:** to determine plane of swelling

Move lump in two directions perpendicular to each other and repeat with the muscle contracted –

- **Skin** (Skin swellings or subjacent swelling fixed to skin): Skin over swelling cannot be pinched
- **Subcutaneous:** Skin can move over lump and lump is free from underlying contracted muscle becomes more prominent when muscle is contracted
- **Muscle:** Lump can be moved sideways but becomes fixed with the contraction of muscle and lump diminished when muscle is contracted
- **Bone:** Immobile even when muscle is relaxed and cannot be moved apart from bone; may disappear with muscle contraction

- <u>Tendon:</u> Moves along with tendon and becomes fixed when muscle is taut against resistance
- <u>Vessels and nerves:</u> Fixed in longitudinal axis of structure and slight mobility in perpendicular axis
- <u>Tear in muscle or tendon:</u> Swelling appears only on muscle contraction

7.   **Pulsatility:** 2 fingers are placed on lump as far apart as possible – it is pulsatile if finger rises with each beat of artery

- <u>Only raised (Transmitted pulsation):</u> Very close to artery
- <u>Raised and separated wide (Expansile pulsation):</u> Arising from artery

8.   **Fluctuation:** Positive in swelling containing liquid or gas; performed in 2 planes right angle to each other

- <u>Fixed lumps:</u> Place 2 fingers on lump as wide apart as possible, press one pole with a finger and feel movement at the other pole
- <u>Freely mobile lumps:</u> Fix and feel with thumb and index finger of 1 hand at 1 pole and press on other pole with thumb and other fingers of the other hand

- <u>Very small lump:</u> Place and feel with 2 fingers in "peace sign" on either edges of the lump and press with index finger of another hand on 1 side of lump
- <u>Very large swelling:</u> More than 1 fingers can be used as "watching" and "displacing" fingers

9. **Irreducibility and compressibility:**

- <u>Reducible:</u> Contents can be completely displaced into cavity (disappears) and may require cough or gravity to reappear (hernia, lymph, varix, varicocele, saphena varix, meningocele, etc.)
- <u>Compressible:</u> Mass decreases with pressure but reappears immediately with release (vascular malformations)

10. **Regional lymph nodes:** Exclude regional lymphadenopathy

11. **Edge/margin:**

- <u>Well defined:</u> Neoplastic and chronic inflammatory swellings
  - Smooth margins (benign growths)
    a. Slip sign: Lipoma
    b. Margin yields to palpating finger: Cysts

- Irregular margins (malignant growths)

- <u>Ill defined:</u> Acute inflammatory swellings

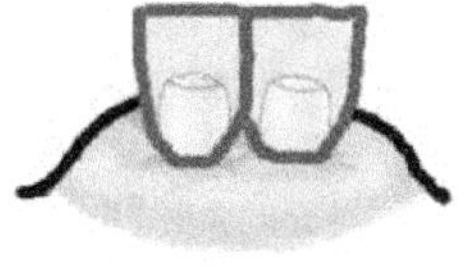

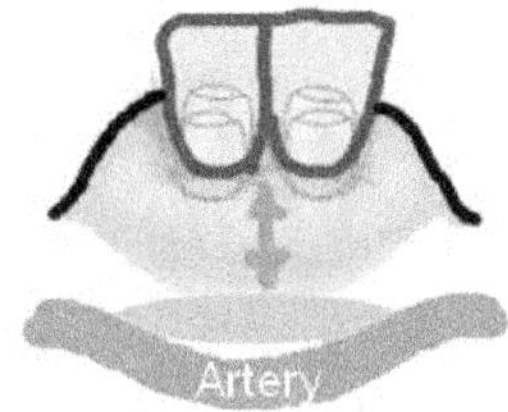

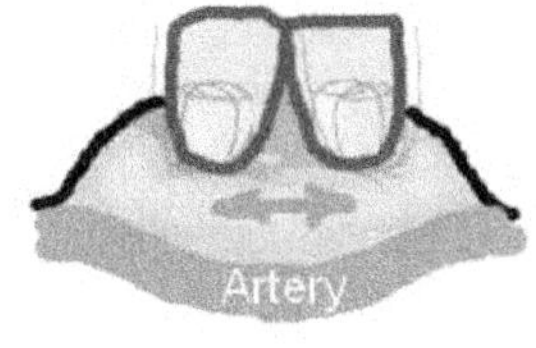

Percussion (Tap)

1. **Tone:** Resonant (gaseous content like hernia, enterocele, pharyngocele) or Dull (solid)

2. **Tinel sign** (positive in schwannoma)

3. **Thrill**

a. <u>Fluid thrill</u> (in swelling containing fluid): Percussion wave is palpable on 1 pole when other pole is tapped

b. <u>Hydatid thrill:</u> middle finger of left hand is placed on the dome of swelling and other 2 adjacent fingers are placed as far apart as possible on the swelling and the right middle finger percusses on the left middle finger and waves are felt on adjacent fingers (displacement of daughter cysts in the fluid of mother cyst)

Auscultation

For pulsatile and peristaltic lumps for bruits/murmurs and bowel sounds

- Bruit: Vascular swellings
- Machinery murmur: Aneurysmal varix
- Bowel sounds: Listen in abdominal and scrotal lumps

Move

Range of motion (ROM) of nearby joints

Measure

To find if there is any wasting proximal or distal to swelling

Completion

1.	**Distal Neurovascular status:** May be involved by pressure effects or encroachment

2.	**General examination:** Lumps may be a cause of consequence of metastasis

- e.g. Breast lumps should prompt an abdominal, respiratory and spinal examination

3.	**Cosmetic and quality of Life:** Establish if the patient is affected by the appearance of lump and whether it affects their quality of life in anyway

Differential diagnoses for a lump

Location	Examples
Skin	Benign: Actinic keratosis, Campbell de Morgan spots, Dermatofibroma, Keratacanthoma, Naevus, Seborrhoeic keratosis
	Malignant: a. Epidermal: BCC, SCC, Melanoma b. Dermal: Dermatofibrosarcoma protuberans (DFSP), Malignant fibrous histiocytoma
Subcutaneous	Cyst
Fat	Lipoma
Artery	Aneurysm
Vein	Varicosity
Nerve	Neuroma
Lymph node	Lymphadenopathy
Muscle	Tumor
Bone	Tumor, Malunited fracture, Osteoma
Others	Ganglion (wrist dorsum), Liver (right hypochondrium), Hernia (groin), etc.

CHAPTER 5

Ulcer Examination

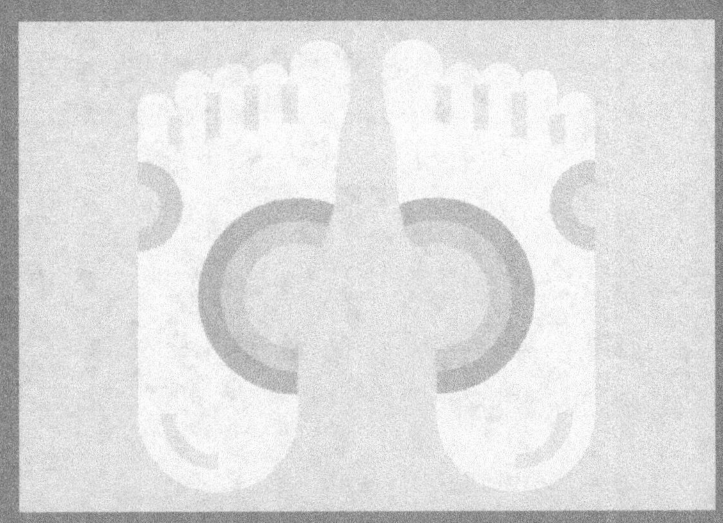

Ulcer Examination

An ulcer is an open sore that results from loss of the epidermis and part or all of the dermis. Ulcers that fail to heal within 6 weeks are defined as chronic. Venous, arterial & neuropathic ulcers are 3 commonest lower extremity ulcers.

Ulcers are clinically examined like Lumps.

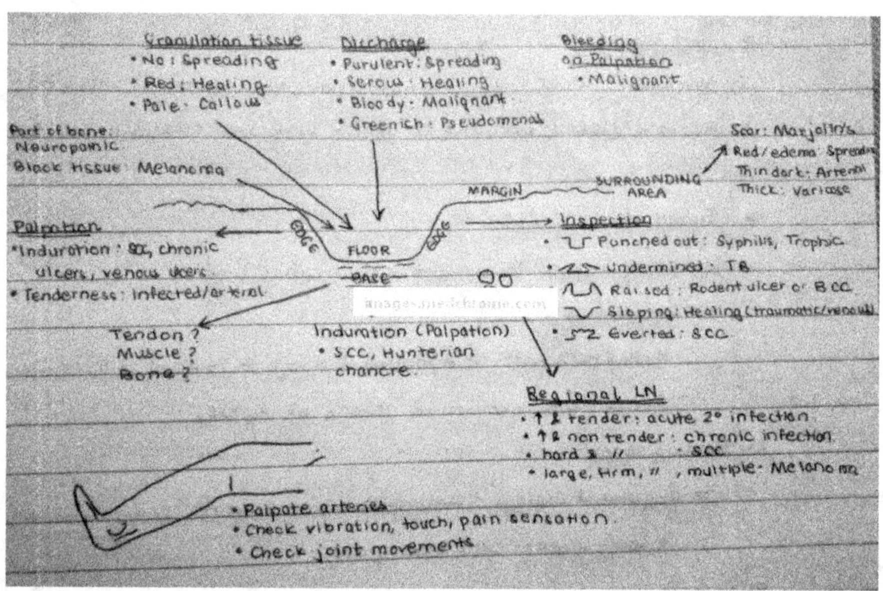

<u>Additional features must be noted:</u>

Mnemonic: Ulcers have **BEDS**

Base = Ulcer rest seat:

- Granulation tissue?/Slough?/Discharge?

Edges and Margins:

1. Margin: Interface among the wall of ulcer & normal epithelium

    i. Sloping: Traumatic and venous ulcers

    ii. Punched: Arterial ulcers

    iii. Undermined: TB

    iv. Rolled: BCC

    v. Everted: SCC, Marjolin's ulcer

2. Edge: Part between margin and floor

Discharge:

1. Purulent: Spreading

2. Serous: Healing

3. Bloody: Malignant

4. Greenish: Pseudomonas

Structures visible (Floor = uncovered ulcer surface):

- Tendon?/Muscle?/Bone?

CHAPTER 6

TL Spine Examination

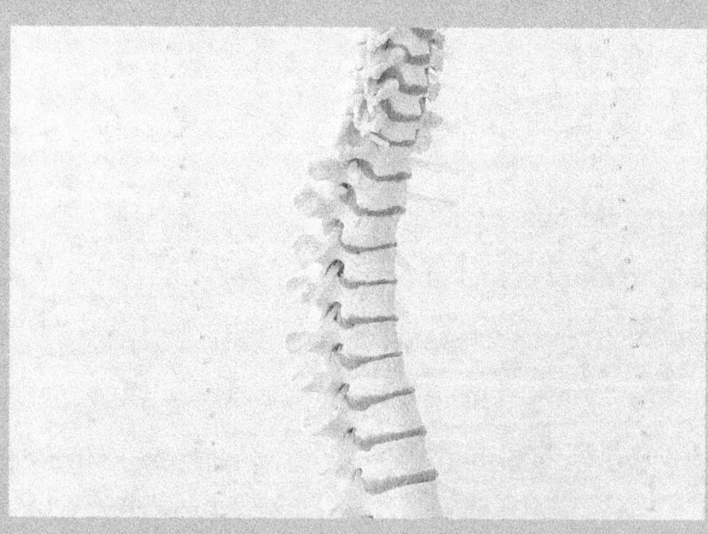

Thoracolumbar Spine Examination

The spine examination involves looking for any deformities, feeling for spinous process tenderness or step-off, recording the spine movements in different planes, special tests like straight leg raise test and performing a complete neurological examination. An assessment should also be made to elicit associated psychological difficulties and any functional impairments.

Exposure

Undress leaving the undergarments only.

Look (Inspection)

Remember the mnemonic **SEADS GO**.

Standing

Ask to stand in Neutral Upright Spinal Alignment (NUSA) position – with the knees and hips comfortably extended, the shoulders and neck neutral

From posterior:

<u>Skin & hair:</u>

- Midline sacral dimple:
    - Simple (<0.5 cm size & <2.5 cm from anal verge & no associated skin abnormalities)
    - Atypical (>0.5 cm size or >2.5 cm from anal verge or associated skin abnormalities) – higher risk of occult spinal dysraphism
    - Tufts of hair: Spinal dysraphism
    - Cafe au lait spots:
        - coast of California (neurofibromatosis): C = smooth = smooth border
        - coast of Maine (McCune Albright): M = ragged = ragged border

- Lumps or bumps

- Erythema or Ecchymosis

- Sinus & Scars

- Hairline & Neck (Short or webbed neck?)

<u>Symmetry:</u> A plumb line can be dropped from C7 to quantify coronal plane deformity –

- Shoulders must be level

- Angle of scapula must be level

- Paraspinal muscles must be symmetrical
  - Spasm (Affected side stands out)
    - Spasm of bilateral muscles may point to serious disease like metastases
    - Wasting (Indicates chronic inflammatory condition like AS or TB or denervation due to previous spinal surgery, poliomyelitis or myopathy)
- PSIS or Iliac crests must be level
  - Pelvic obliquity may be due to:
    - Scoliosis

- - Limb length discrepancy (LLD)
- List (abrupt planar shift of the spine, above a certain point, to one side):
  - Herniated lumbar disc
    - Towards painful side (disc protrusion lies medial to nerve root, i.e. at the axilla)
    - Away from painful side (disc protrusion lies lateral to nerve root, i.e. at the shoulder)
    - Alternating deviation (dura slips from one side to another over a small midline protrusion)
    - Deviation with flexion but not in standing (root pain)
    - Momentary deviation during flexion (fragment of disc alters its position & temporarily touches duramater)
- Step-off deformity
  - Severe grades of spondylolisthesis
- Marked wasting of calves, hamstrings or buttocks:
  - L5 or S1 palsy

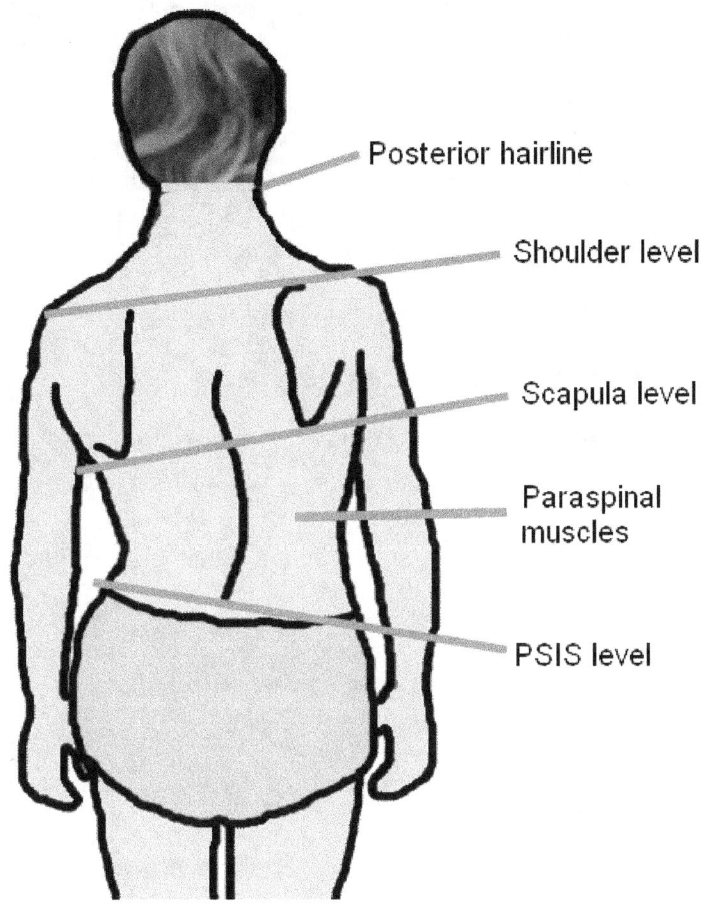

From Lateral:

Kyphosis: Average thoracic kyphosis is 20-45°

- Cervico-thoracic junction: Ankylosing spondylitis
- Thoracic region:
    - Scheuermann's disease

- Multiple osteoporotic vertebral fractures

Hyperlordosis (swayback): Average lumbar lordosis is 40-60°

- Flexion deformities at hip
- High grade spondylolisthesis
- Below primary thoracic kyphotic deformity

Decreased lordosis:

- Muscle spasm (PIVD, Infection)
- Ankylosing spondylitis

Complete loss of lordosis (Flat back syndrome):

- Anterior wedge compression fractures of lumbar vertebrae
- Advanced degeneration of lumbar vertebral discs
- Long thoraco-lumbar spinal fusions

Angular kyphosis

- Pott's spine
- Vertebral body collapse due to tumors, other infections or fractures

Reduction of the space between iliac crest & thoracic cage:

- Shortening of thoracolumbar spine (disc space narrowing at consecutive levels or severe osteoporosis)

Prominent buttocks, shortened trunk, flexed hips & knees: Severe disc slips

From anterior:

- Level of shoulders
- Position of head on shoulders
- Shape of chest:
    - Rib prominence (hump) in Scoliosis
    - Pectus carinatum
    - Pectus excavatum

Bending forwards

Ask to bend forwards (Adam's forward bend) - Look for rib prominence (structural scoliosis)

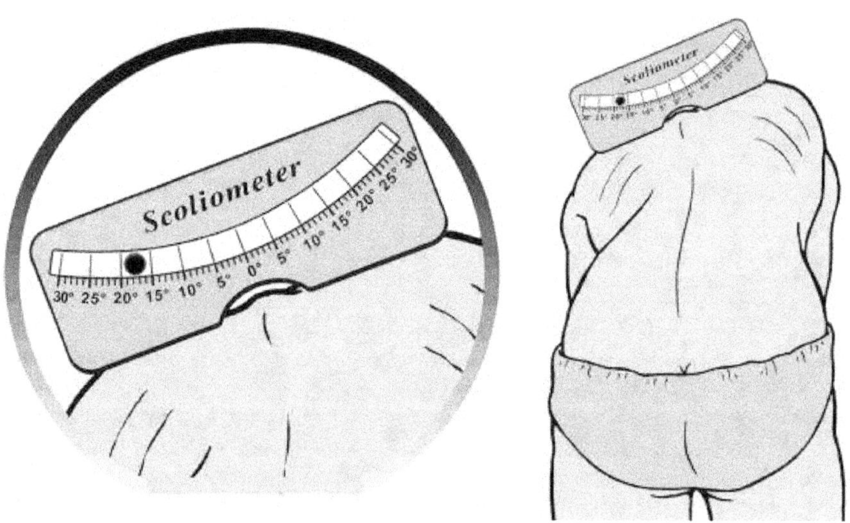

Persistence of deformity as a rib prominence on Adam's test indicate Structural scoliosis

Bending sidewards

Ask to bend sidewards if scoliosis:

- To assess flexibility of curve

Feel (Palpation)

Palpation of the spine is confined to the posterior aspect. Remember the mnemonic **TEST Areas**.

Superficial

a. Local temperature

b. Superficial tenderness:

- Positive in skin conditions
- <u>Pinch skin folds:</u> Widespread superficial tenderness may indicate functional overlay (Wadell's sign)

Deep

a. Paraspinal muscles: Optimal site of palpation is approximately 2 inches from midline

- Spasm: Ask to bend towards the affected side (expected to soften and relax but remains firm in spasm)
- Trigger points and tender nodules: Fibromyalgia

b. Spinous process and Interspinous spaces:

- <u>Identify & mark landmarks (as a reference for counting up & down):</u> May vary by 1 vertebral level
  —
    - Line through top of iliac crests (Intercristal line or Tuffier's line) = L4/L5 interspace
    - Line through top of PSIS (dimple at midline or dimple of venus) = S2
    - Most prominent spinous process at base of neck = T1
    - Line through inferior angle of scapula = T7
- <u>Tenderness:</u>
    - Direct pressure tenderness:
        - Any pathology in spinous process
        - Advanced pathology in vertebral body
    - Rotatory or Twist tenderness: twist side of spinous process using thumb

- Any pathology in spinous process
- Early pathology in vertebral body
- Thrust tenderness (Percussion tenderness): gentle thumping with ulnar border of fist (if above 2 methods have failed to elicit tenderness)
- <u>Step off (when running fingers down the midline of spine):</u> Spondylolisthesis (palpable usually from Meyerding's Grade III)
- <u>Interspinous space width & tenderness</u>

e. Facet joints: On each side of spinous processes

f. Iliac crests and PSIS

g. Sacroiliac joints (SIJ): 1 inch medial and 1 inch inferior to PSIS

- <u>Tenderness:</u> Sacroiliac strain or Sacroiliitis

h. Sacro-coccygeal junction:

- <u>Tenderness:</u> Coccydynia

Move (Range of Motion)

Move	ROM	Instruction	Assessment Methods
Flexion	80-90°	Attempt to touch floor with fingertips/palms with knee extended	a. Angle between final position of trunk & a vertical plane b. Fingertip to floor distance: normally 0-20 cm c. Position of fingers reaching leg (eg. tibia shin, knee, etc.) d. Schober's test (lumbar spine): increase in distance between 2 points (midpoint of line joining 2 PSIS and a point 10 cm above it) by ≥5 cm

			e. Modified Schober's test (lumbar spine): increase in distance between 2 points (5 cm below inter-PSIS midpoint and 10 cm above inter-PSIS midpoint) by ≥5 cm (greater distance reduces the range of error) f. Ott's test or Thoracic schober test (thoracic spine): increase in distance between 2 points (C7 spinous process and a point 12 inches/30 cm distal to it) ≥8 cm
Extend	20-30°	Place both hands on iliac crest (to stabilize pelvis) & lean backward as far as possible	a. Angle between trunk & vertical line b. Distance decreased between L1 and S1 can also be measured (normally ≥1-2 cm)

Lateral bend	30-40°	The examiner stabilizes the patient's pelvis with a hand on each iliac crest and asks the standing patient to lean as far as possible to each side	a. Angle between trunk (imaginary line between C7-S1) & vertical line b. Position of fingertips reaching the leg (knee, upper leg, etc.)
Rotate (hips anchored by examiner or in sitting position with arms folded on chest)	30-40°	Rotate or twist in each direction as far as possible	Angle between inter-acromial line and inter-ASIS line

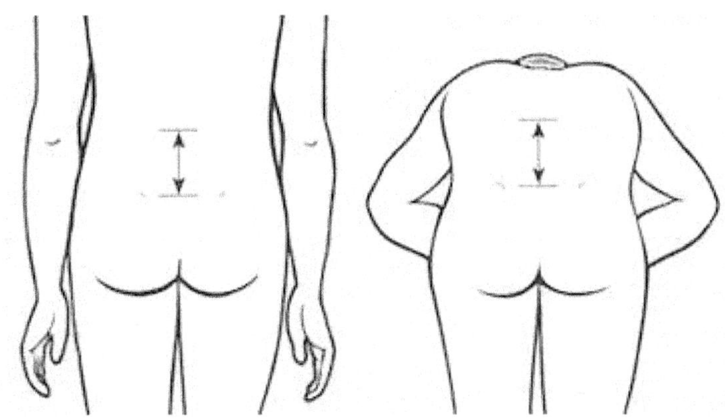

Schober's test for measuring lumbar flexion
Nasch92, CC BY-SA 4.0, via Wikimedia Commons

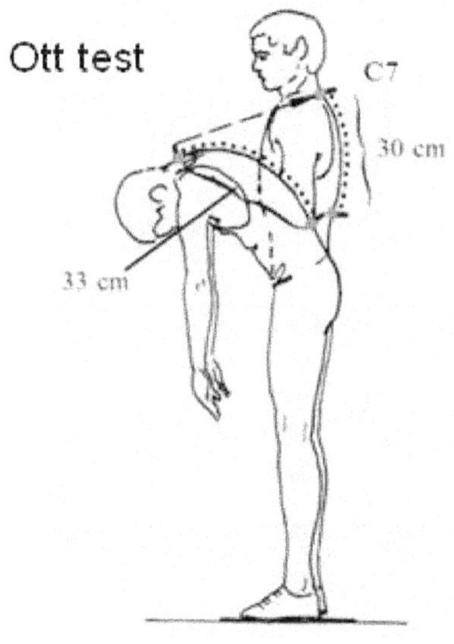

Move	Interpretation
Flexion	Decreased: a. Disc prolapse b. Ankylosing spondylitis c. Hamstring shortening d. Short paravertebral muscles (spasm) e. Decreased hip joint motion Increased: Generalized hypermobility
Extension	Decreased: 1. Facet joint arthrosis 2. Disc protrusions 3. Arched sacrum 4. Baastrup's disease (kissing spine) 5. Hip problems

Lateral bending	Decreased: a. On the convex side of scoliosis b. Muscle contractions c. Disc protrusions on same side d. Ankylosing spondylosis e. SIJ lesions f. Hip joint pathology

Measure

1. **Pelvic obliquity:** Angle between Inter-crest or Inter-ASIS line and horizontal

2. **Sciatic list:** Horizontal distance between C7 plumb line and CSVL (Central sacral vertical line)

3. **Iliocostal distance (Rib-pelvis distance):** Distance between inferior margin of ribs and superior edge of iliac crest in mid-axillary line in finger-breadths or centimeters

- Normal: >2 finger-breadth
- Unilateral decrease: Convex side of scoliosis

- Bilateral decreased: Kyphosis due to occult lumbar vertebral fractures

- Iliocostal contact may cause Iliocostal friction syndrome or costo-iliac impingement

4. **Wall-occiput distance:** Distance between wall and occiput when patient is asked to stand on wall touching the occiput and heels to the wall (>0 is considered positive for kyphosis due to occult thoracic vertebral fractures)

5. **Chest expansion:** At expiration and maximum inspiration measured at nipple line, i.e. T4-T5

- <2.5 cm is considered abnormal
- Gauzes costo-vertebral movement

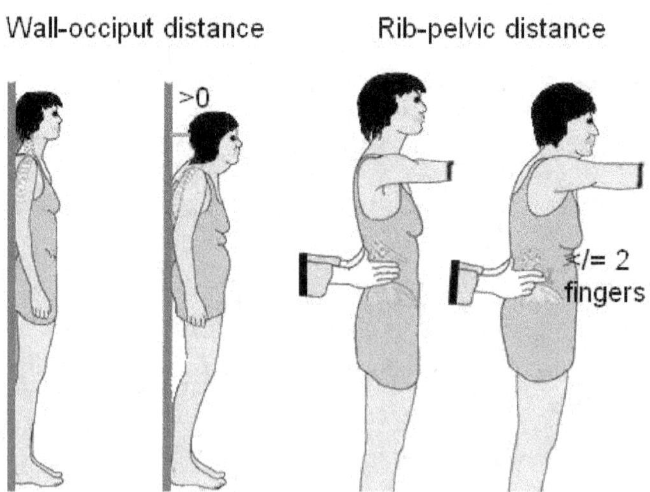

Screen (Before Walk)

1. Romberg test (Dorsal column/Proprioception)

2. Squat and get up (L3)

3. Stand on heels (L4)

4. Stand on one leg/Trendelenburg test (L5)

5. Stand on tiptoes (S1)

Walk (Gait)

1. **With hip more extended & knee more flexed (to relieve tension from sciatic nerve):** Sciatica
2. **Antalgic gait:** Lumbar radiculopathy secondary to disc prolapse
3. **Trendelenburg gait:** Injury to L5 nerve root
4. **High steppage gait (foot drop):** Injury to common peroneal nerve or sciatic nerve
5. **Short limb gait:** Scoliosis leading to compensatory LLD

Neurovascular Examination

1. Higher functions (assess at time of history taking):
consciousness, alertness, orientation, speech

2. Motor:

- Bulk
- Tone (Modified Ashworth scale)
  epomedicine.com/clinical-medicine/modified-ash
  worth-scale-for-spasticity-mnemonic/
- Power
- Coordination (heel-shin test, finger nose test)
- Involuntary movements

3. Reflex:

- **Superficial**
  - Abdominal (T7-12)
  - Cremasteric (L1-2)
  - Plantar response (L5,S1)

- Beevor's sign -

    https://epomedicine.com/clinical-medicine/beevors-sign/

- **Deep**

    - Knee jerk (L3,L4)

    - Medial hamstring (L5)

    - Ankle (S1)

    - Clonus (patellar, ankle): Sustained = >5 beats

    https://epomedicine.com/clinical-medicine/deep-tendon-reflexes/

4. **Sensory:**

- **Superficial:**

    - Pain (pin prick)

    - Fine touch (wisp of cotton)

    - Temperature (test tubes containing hot and cold water or tuning fork)

- **Deep:**

    - Joint position sense

    - Vibration sense (128 Hz tuning fork)

- **Cortical:**
  - 2 point discrimination
  - Stereognosis

ROOT	MOTOR	SENSORY	REFLEX
L2	Iliopsoas (Resisted hip flexion)	Mid-anterior thigh	None
L3	Quadriceps (Resisted knee extension)	Medial femoral condyle	Patellar
L4	Tibialis anterior (Resisted ankle dorsiflexion and inversion)	Medial malleolus	Patellar
L5	Extensor hallucis longus and Extensor digitorum longus (Resisted great-toe dorsiflexion); Resisted ankle eversion; Gluteus medius (abduction)	1st web space	Hamstring or Semitendinosus reflex
S1	Tendo-achilles, Flexor hallucis longus, Flexor digitorum longus (Resisted ankle plantar flexion)	Lateral plantar foot	Achilles

Posterolateral disc protrusions will impinge on traversing nerve root (L4/L5 PIVD - L5 nerve root). Far lateral disc protrusions will impinge on exiting nerve root (L4/L5 PIVD - L4 nerve root).

5. **Sudomotor examination:**

- Stroke the skin with finger or barrel of pen: pulls smoothly over dry (symathectomized) skin but irregularly and unevenly over normal moist skin

6. **All peripheral pulses:**

- Vascular claudication can mimic radiculopathy & spinal canal stenosis

Provocative tests for Lumbar spine

Standing

1. **Quadrant test or Kemp's test:** Assist the patient in extending the spine maximally holding the shoulders,

then ask patient to rotate and lateral flex to the site of pain –

- Symptoms more concordant to those of neurogenic claudication: Lumbar spinal stenosis
- Pain predominant: Facet joint arthrosis

2. **Stork test:** Extension of spine standing on one leg, then clinician passively hyper-extends and rotates the patient towards weight bearing side

- Pain reproduction: Spondylolysis and possible spondylolisthesis

Supine

1. **Straight leg raising test (SLRT) or Lasegue's test and sensitizers (Sciatic nerve):**

- 0-30 degrees – Tone the slack
- 30-70 degrees – Sliding and stretching
- 70-90 degrees – Only stretching
- Sensitizers:
  - Passive dorsiflexion of the foot (Braggard's test)

- ○ Applying firm pressure to lateral popliteal nerve behind the lateral tibial condyle, to tighten it like a bowstring (Bowstring test)
- ○ Passive cervical flexion (Soto-Hall test)

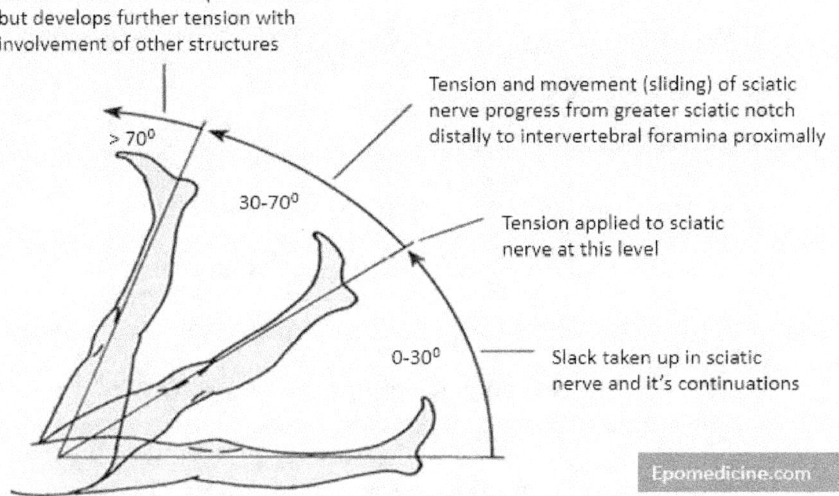

https://epomedicine.com/medical-students/straight-leg-raising-test-pathophysiology/

2. **Well's crossed leg SLRT (Fajersztajn test):** more specific; may indicate large paracentral disc herniation

3. **Hoover's test (for functional weakness):** The patient is unable to extend the hip and to press the heel into the

bed on request. The hip is extended involuntarily when the opposite leg is lifted off the bed.

Sitting

1. **Bechtrew's test (seated SLR):** can be undertaken as a part of flip test (Waddel's sign)

2. **Slump test:** ask the patient to flex spine (slump), followed by passive neck flexion, active knee extension and dorsiflexion of foot (positive nerve root tension sign if pain) and relieved on returning neck to neutral

3. **Tripod sign:** passively extend the patient's knee (patient will lean backwards with support of hands or slump forwards in hamstring contractures)

4. **Naffziger's test:** Jugular compression leading to pain in lumbar region suggests intrathecal space occupying lesion in lumbar region (can also use Valsalva maneuver)

Prone

Femoral nerve stretch test (for L3-L4): Flex the patient's knee and lifting the hip into extension – pain may be elicited down the front of the thigh

Waddel's sign

Waddell identified 5 exam findings that correlated with non-organic low back pain. The tests include

1. Tenderness:
     - Superficial – pain with light touch to skin
     - Deep – nonanatomic widespread deep pain
2. Simulation:
     - Pain with light axial compression on skull
     - Pain with light twisting of pelvis
3. Distraction
     - No pain with distracted SLR
4. Regional disturbance:
     - Nonanatomic or inconsistent motor findings during entire exam
     - Nonanatomic or inconsistent sensory findings during entire exam
5. Overreaction
     - Overreaction noted at any time during exam

Completion

1. **Tests for Sacro-iliac joint** (Distraction test - best for screening):
     - The examiner places the hands on the ASIS with the arms crossed

- Pressure is exerted in a downward and outward direction and should be evenly distributed to prevent moving the lumbar region
- Positive: Unilateral pain in gluteal region

2. **Tests for Hip joint**
    - ROM (with end-feel & pain if present)

3. **Per-rectal examination (for S3, S4, S5):**
    - Resting and active motor function of external anal sphincter
    - Anal sensation
    - Bulbocavernosus reflex
        1. tests for the presence of spinal shock
        2. positive reflex with anal sphincter contraction with squeezing of glans penis or clitorus (or tug foley catheter)

CHAPTER 7

Hip Examination

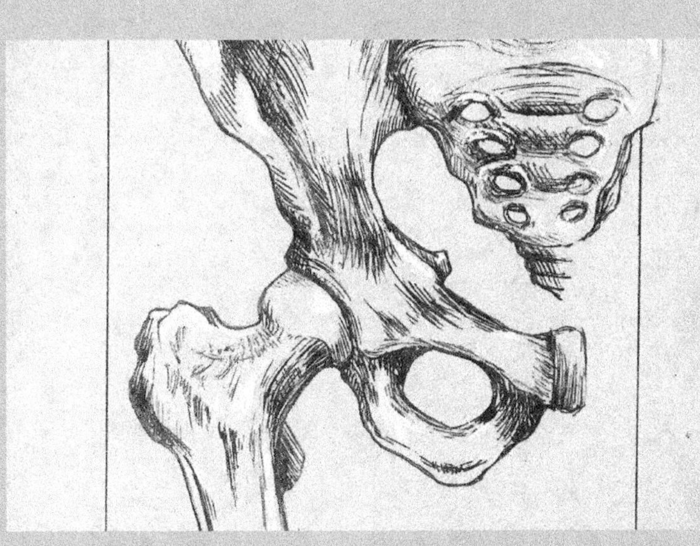

Hip Examination

The hip examination should evaluate the hip, back, abdomen, and vascular and neurologic systems. This chapter is adapted from the 21 steps hip examination proposed by Hal David Martin and Ian James Palmer. Besides the joint, clinician must be cognizant of bone problems, surrounding musculotendinous and bursal structures, neurological disorders and visceral problems that have potential to refer to pain in the hip area.

Standing

1. **Note general point of pain:** C sign (Patients with intra-articular hip pathology often localize the area of pain by cupping the thumb and index finger in the shape of the letter C)

2. **Gait (Watch 6-8 stride lengths):** Pelvic tilt/rotation, Stride length, Stance phase, FPA

https://epomedicine.com/clinical-medicine/physical-examination-gait/

3. **Single leg stance phase test:** This test is positive in conditions in which any of the three – fulcrum (femoral head), lever arm (femoral neck length) or power (muscles/nerves) are affected. It can be remembered using the mnemonic: **Sound Side Sags**.

https://epomedicine.com/clinical-medicine/trendelenburg-test-or-sign/

4. **Inspection:**

- Body habitus
- Spinal alignment: Shoulder-iliac crest heights, lordosis, scoliosis (towards affected side in abduction deformity, towards normal side in adduction deformity; hint: side wherever ASIS is lower) , leg length (tilted pelvis, equinus on shorter side, knee flexion on longer side)
- Symmetry of gluteal folds: Asymmetrical on developmental dysplasia of hip, muscular dystrophy or leg length discrepancy
- Forward bending (Structural vs Nonstructural scoliosis; ROM) and lateral bending ROM
- Laxity: Beighton scale

Seated

5. **Vascular and Lymphatic examination:** Dorsalis pedis and posterior tibial artery pulse; Skin for swelling, scarring or side-to-side asymmetry

6. **Neurologic:** Sensory and Motor function and DTR (Patellar, Achilles)

7. **Passive straight leg raise:** Radicular neurologic symptoms

8. **Passive hip rotation:** Seated position ensures that the ischium is square to the table, thus providing adequate stability at 90 degrees of hip flexion

- <u>Internal rotation:</u> Normal 20-35 degrees
- <u>External rotation:</u> Normal 30-45 degrees

Supine

9. Inspect for leg length discrepancies (LLD)

10. **Palpate:**

- Bony landmarks: ASIS, Iliac crest, Greater trochanter, Symphysis pubis, Pubic tubercle, Adductor tubercle
- Local temperature
- Joint tenderness:
    - <u>Anteriorly:</u> 2 cm below and lateral to mid-inguinal point
    - <u>Posteriorly:</u> Junction of lateral 1/3 and medial 2/3 of a line joining GT and PSIS
- Vascular sign of Narath (Femoral pulse)
- Inguinal lymph nodes
- Abdomen

11. **Range of Motion: Flexion, abduction, adduction**

Movement	Norm al (°)	Center	Stationary arm	Moving arm
Seated internal rotation	20-35	Center of patella	Aligned vertically	Line to tibial crest and midway between malleoli

Seated external rotation	30-45	Center of patella	Aligned vertically	Line to tibial crest and midway between malleoli
Extended internal rotation	20-35	Center of patella	Aligned horizontally	Line to tibial crest and midway between malleoli
Extended external rotation	30-45	Center of patella	Aligned horizontally	Line to tibial crest and midway between malleoli
Supine hip flexion	100-110	GT	Lateral midline of pelvis	Line to lateral femoral epicondyle
Adduction	20-30	ASIS	Line to other ASIS	Line to midline patella
Abduction	45	<45	Line to other ASIS	Line to midline patella

Further details on goniometric assessment:

http://at.uwa.edu/gon/hip.htm

Sectoral sign: If the range of motion for rotation varies between 2 positions by 20 degrees, it is considered as differential rotation. In the osteonecrosis of the hip, there is positive differential rotation of the hip in flexion compared to the extension which is called a sectoral sign.

https://epomedicine.com/clinical-medicine/sectoral-sign-avn-hip/

12. **Fixed adduction and abduction deformity:**

- ASIS at both sides at same level: Pelvis square
- ASIS at affected side higher: Fixed adduction deformity
- ASIS at affected side lower: Fixed abduction deformity
- Squaring of pelvis: Bring the ASIS into same level by further adducting in adduction deformity and abducting in the abduction deformity
- Quantifying the fixed adduction and abduction deformity:
    - Squaring the pelvis: Angle of adduction or abduction with the vertical line

- ■ <u>Kothari's angle:</u> A line is drawn from suprasternal notch to symphysis pubis. Perpendicular is dropped from ASIS to this line and the angle between this line and the line connecting the ASIS on two sides form the Kothari's angle.

13. Thomas test

- Patient lies supine with knee against chest position on the "good" side until lumbar lordosis disappears

- One hand is placed behind the lumbar spine to assess the degree of lumbar lordosis.

- If there is no lordosis when the affected limb lies flat on the couch there can be no fixed flexion deformity and there is no need to proceed with the test.

- The examiner then passively presses down on the affected side thigh until ASIS begins to move forward. The angle of the thigh to the bed is the angle of fixed flexion deformity (FFD).

- **Further reading:**

  https://epomedicine.com/clinical-medicine/thom
  as-test/

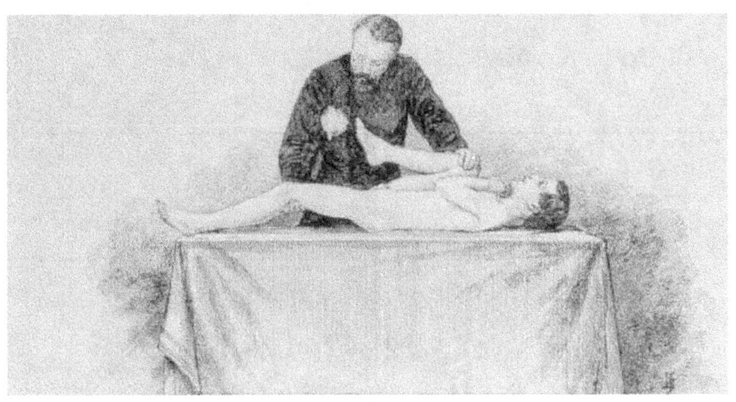

Hugh Owen Thomas, CC BY-SA 4.0, via Wikimedia Commons

14. FADIR (Flexion, Adduction, Internal rotation):

- <u>Hip pain:</u> Anterior femoroacetabular impingement, Torn labrum

- <u>Pain along the piriformis distribution or sciatic nerve pain down the leg:</u> Piriformis syndrome

15. FABER (Flexion, Abduction, External rotation; Patrick test; Figure of 4 position): Distinguish between back and hip pathology, specifically sacroiliac joint

- <u>Sacoiliac discomfort:</u> Sacroiliitis

- <u>Recreation of hip pain:</u> Posterior femoroacetabular impingement, ligamentous injury or trochanteric pathologies

16. DIRI test and DEXRIT

DIRI test	DEXRIT
Dynamic internal rotation impingement test	Dynamic external rotation impingement test
Establish 0 pelvic set point & eliminate lumbar lordosis by holding non-affected leg in flexion beyond 90° – examined hip is brought into 90° of flexion or beyond & is passively taken through a wide arc of adduction & internal rotation	Establish 0 pelvic set point & eliminate lumbar lordosis by holding non-affected leg in flexion beyond 90° – examined hip is brought into 90° of flexion or beyond & is passively taken through a wide arc of abduction and external rotation
Positive – Hip pain	Positive – Hip pain
Anterior FAI, torn labrum	Superior FAI, torn labrum

17. **Posterior rim impingement test (EABER; Extension, Abduction, External rotation):** Posterior FAI, torn labrum

The patient is positioned at the edge or end of the examination table so that the leg can hang freely to full extension. The patient established the pelvic zero set-point with both legs held in flexion. The examined leg is allowed to reach full extension off the table, and then taken into abduction and external rotation.

18. **Passive supine rotation (log roll) test:**

Gently roll the limb into internal rotation and external rotation. Pain suggests intra-articular hip pathology.

Dial test: Passive internal rotation of the leg, followed by releasing the leg and allowing it to external rotate. External rotation of more than contralateral limb or more than 45°, relative to vertical, is a positive test and indicates iliofemoral ligament laxity.

19. Heel strike: Trauma or femoral fracture

20. Straight leg raise against resistance (to 45 degrees;
Stinchfield test): Pain (intra-articular pathology as the
iliopsoas presses against the acetabular labrum during
active resistance) or Iliopsoas weakness

21. **Length measurements:**

- Apparent length measurement: Place the legs
  parallel; Midline point of body (xiphisternum or
  umbilicus) to tip of medial malleolus (adduction
  makes the limb appear shorter – each 10 degrees
  of fixed adduction/abduction add a further 3 cm
  change in apparent length to any real shortening)
- True length measurement: Place the normal limb
  in a comparable position of adduction or
  abduction to the abnormal limb; ASIS to medial
  malleolus (if there is a fixed deformity, the good
  leg must be placed in a comparable deformed
  position relative to the pelvis)
- Is the shortening above or below the knee
  a. Segmental measurements: Measure –
      - Femur: from ASIS to medial knee
        joint line

- Tibia: from medial knee joint line to tip of medial malleolus

b. <u>Galeazzi's test</u>: If both knees are flexed while the heels remain together on the couch, it can be seen whether the shortening is in the femur or tibia.

- Knee lies lower down: Tibial shortening
- Knee lies proximally: Femoral shortening

- If the shortening is in femur, is it <u>above the trochanter or below the trochanter?</u>

a. Bryant's triangle: Not helpful in bilateral hip joint pathology

b. Chiene's parallelogram: 2 lines joining the GT on both sides and ASIS on both sides must be parallel (supratrochanteric shortening at 1 side leads to convergence of line)

c. Schoemaker's line: The lines passing through GT to ASIS on both sides normally meets in the midline above the umbilicus

- Unilateral supratrochanteric shortening: Meet away from the midline on opposite side
- Bilateral supratrochanteric shortening: Meet in midline but inferior to umbilicus

- <u>Interpretation of shortening:</u>
    a. True shortening = Apparent shortening: No compensation
    b. True shortening > Apparent shortening: Partial compensation with Fixed abduction deformity
    c. True shortening < Apparent shortening: Fixed adduction deformity without compensation

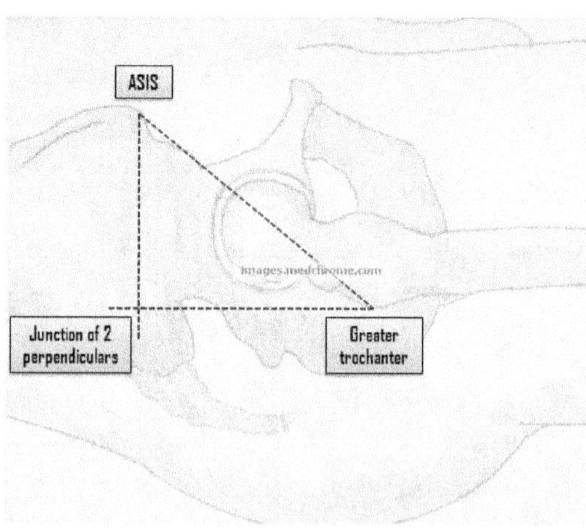

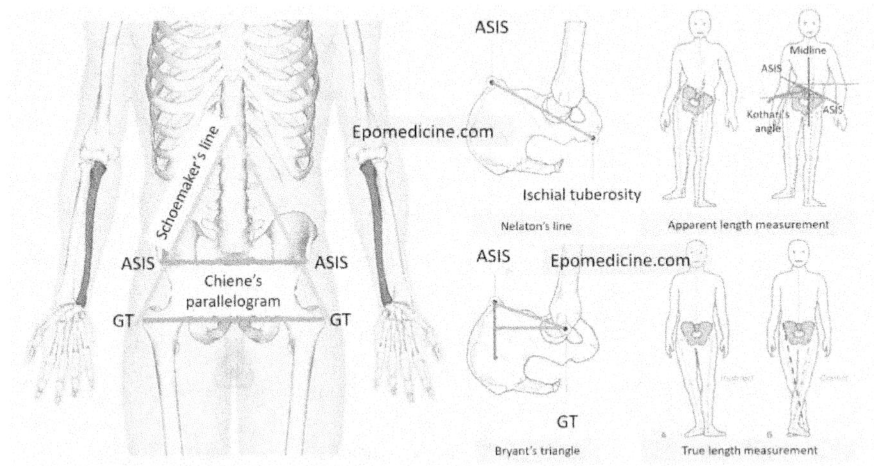

Schoemaker's line – Line through ASIS & GT on both side must meet in center at or above umbilicus; **Chiene's parallelogram** – Line through ASIS on both sides must be parallel to line through GT on both sides; **Nelaton's line** – GT lies on or below the line through GT to ischial tuberosity when the hip is flexed to 90°; **Bryant's triangle** – Base of the triangle compared on both sides (between a perpendicular dropped from ASIS and the hypotenuse between ASIS and GT); **Morris' bitrochanteric test:** distance between GT & pubic symphysis on both sides; **Apparent length measurement** – Both limbs are kept parallel & measurement is done from umbilicus/xiphisternum to medial malleolus; **True length measurement** (done if apparent shortening present) – Normal limb is kept identical to limb with abduction or adduction deformity if present and measurement done from ASIS to medial malleolus; **Kothari's angle** – Abduction and adduction deformity can be quantified using an angle formed by a line connecting ASIS on both sides and the perpendiculars dropped from ASIS to midline

https://epomedicine.com/clinical-medicine/bryants-triangle/

22. **Telescopic test:** Stabilize the pelvis by pressing on ASIS with thumb and thenar eminence of one hand while the fingertips touch the greater trochanter. Flex the affected hip & knee to 90° & grasp the distal thigh & knee between your chest & right armpit. Push & pull along the longitudinal axis of the femur. Note the amount of excursion of the tip of the trochanter with fingertips and compare to the opposite side. It may be positive in:

- Nonunion neck of femur
- Old unreduced posterior dislocation of hip
- DDH
- Pathological dislocation of hip
- Girdlestone arthroplasty
- Septic sequelae of hip

Lateral

23. **Palpation:**

- Supra-sacroiliac area, SI joint, gluteus maximus origin, piriformis muscle
- Facets of greater trochanter (gluteus minimus inserts at anterior facet, gluteus medius inserts at posterosuperior and lateral facet, trochanteric bursa at posterior facet)
- Sciatic nerve (Sciatic point): midway between ischial tuberosity & posterior border of trochanter with hip flexed (moves gluteus maximus away)
    - **Tenderness:** Herniated lumbar disc, Spasm of piriformis, Direct trauma over nerve

24. **Abductor strength:**

- <u>Overall:</u> With knee in extension
- <u>Gluteus medius:</u> With knee in flexion (to release gluteus maximus contribution for the ITB)
- <u>Gluteus maximus:</u> Abducting and extending the hip

25. **Ober's test:**

Patient lies laterally on the normal side with hip & knee flexed (for stability and to flatten the lumbar curve). The examiner stabilizes the pelvis/greater trochanter with one hand. With the other hand, the knee is flexed to 90°. The examiner then gradually lifts (abducts & extends the hip to center the ITB on greater trochanter) of the affected leg with the knee flexed. Then, the examiner slowly allows the upper leg to lower down (making sure the hip doesn't fall into flexion & internal rotation) until the examiner is no longer supporting the weight of the upper leg. With **tight TFL & ITB,** the affected leg would remain in an abducted position & doesn't fall to the table or the pelvis tilts laterally & the patient experiences lateral knee pain.

https://epomedicine.com/clinical-medicine/obers-test/

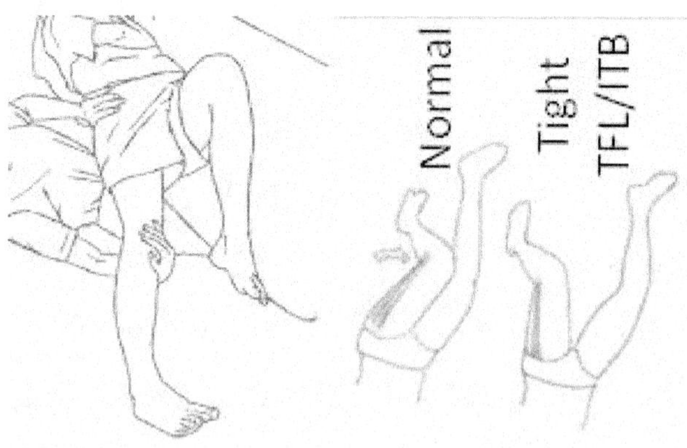

26. **Ischiofemoral impingement test (HEADER; Hip extension, abduction, external rotation)**

27. **Nelaton's line:** A measuring tape of string is stretched from ischial tuberosity to ASIS with hip in 90 degrees flexion. Normally, the greater trochanter lies on or below the line. If the trochanter lies above the line, this indicates that the femur has migrated proximally.

Prone

28. **Palpate:**

   - Gluteus maximus: Hip extended, and buttocks squeezed together

29. **Range of motion:** Test extension of hip, flexing the knee (relaxes hamstrings) – around 30 degrees

31. **Prone hip extension (Staheli) test:** Patient lies prone on the edge of the table. The examiner places one hand on the pelvis and gradually extends the thigh with the other. The point at which the pelvis begins to rise indicates the end of hip motion and beginning of

movement at the spine. At this point, the horizontal-thigh angle is measured. It can be used for bilateral hip pathology.

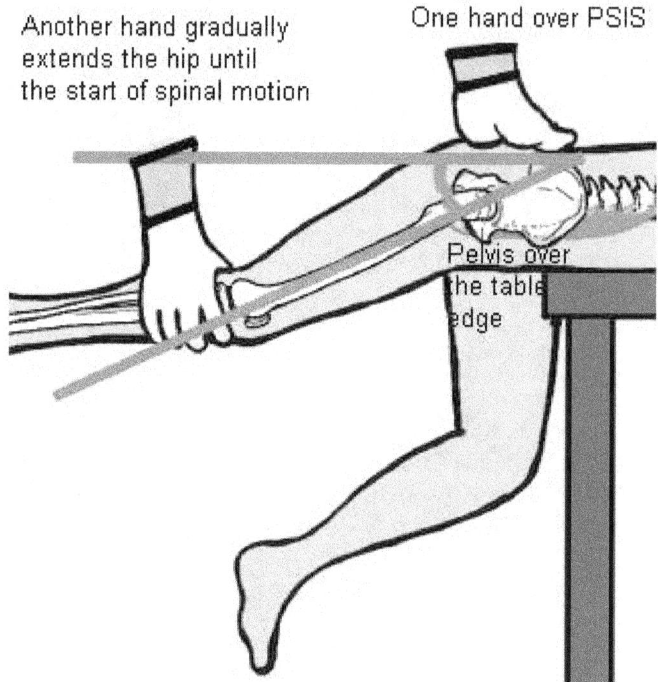

Staheli's Prone extension test

32. **Ely's test:**

Patient is positioned prone. With one hand of the examiner on the patient's lower back, the other hand holds the patient's leg at heel and flexes the knee towards the buttocks making sure the leg doesn't abduct.

<u>Positive test</u>: When the patient is unable to flex or touch the heels towards the buttocks and the hip of the affected side rises up from the table, the patient will also feel or complain of pain or tingling in the back or legs indicates a positive Ely's test.

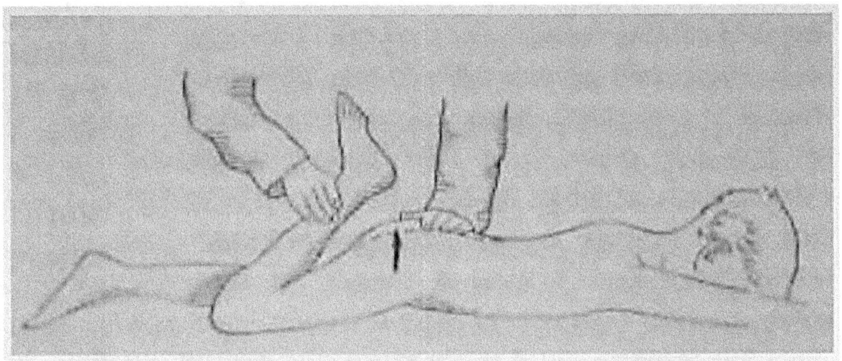

- The **Duncan-ely** test: patient is positioned prone. As the knee is flexed, a contracture of the rectus femoris causes the hip to flex because rectus femoris is a hip flexor and knee extensor.

33. Craig's test:

Patient lies prone with knee on the test side flexed to 90 degrees. Examiner palpates the greater trochanter and internally and externally rotates the hip until the greater trochanter lies at the lateral most aspect of the hip (the greater trochanter is parallel to the examination table or bed at this point) thereby projecting the femoral head into center of acetabulum.

<u>Angle measurement:</u> Measure the angle of internal or external rotation using the goniometer.

<u>Interpretation:</u>

- Normal: At birth, the mean anteversion angle is 30 degrees which decreases to 8-15 degrees in adults (angle of internal rotation).
- Angle >15 degrees: Increased anteversion leads to squinting patellae & pigeon toed walking (in-toeing) which is twice as common in girls.
- Angle <8 degrees: Retroversionenter of acetabulum.

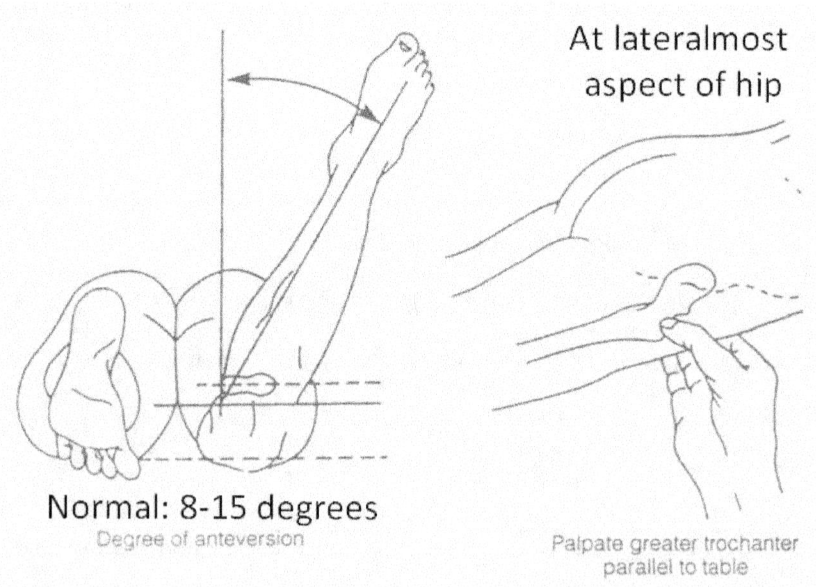

34. **Phelp's test (gracilis tightness):** Affected hip is abducted as far as possible; the knee is then flexed over the side of the couch. If more abduction is possible by flexing the knee (and relaxing the gracilis), then this signifies that the gracilis is tight.

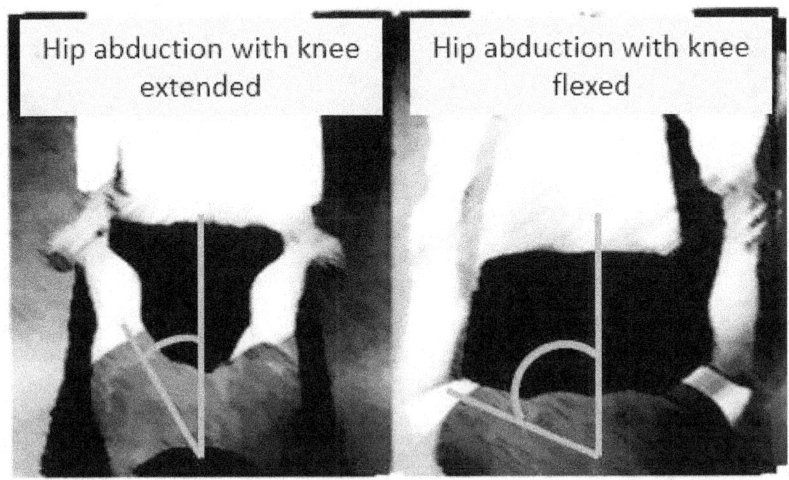

CHAPTER 8

Knee Examination

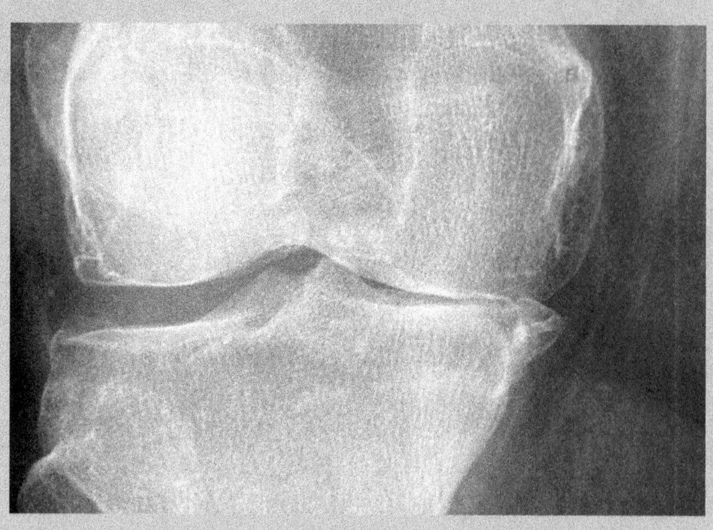

Knee Examination

Knee as a joint is a complex structure consisting of bones, ligaments, menisci and surrounding musculotendinous and bursal structures. The clinical examination of a knee is performed to evaluate three aspects: 1) Patellofemoral joint/Extensor mechanism; 2) Articular (meniscal and chondral) lesions; and 3) Knee instability.

Exposure

From flanks to ankle

Look (Inspection)

On inspection, remember the mnemonic **SEADS GO**.

Standing

a. From anterior:

<u>Knee alignment:</u>

- o Q-angle (Quadriceps angle): Angle between a line drawn from ASIS to Center of patella & Tibial tuberosity to Center of patella
    - M: 8-14°
    - F: 15-17°
    - Abnormal ≥20°

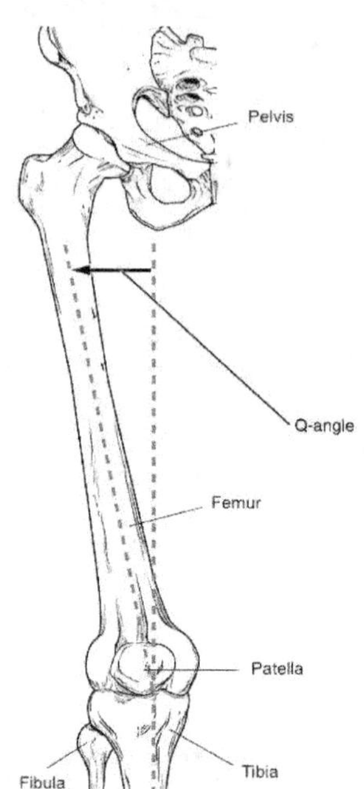

OpenStax College, CC BY-SA 4.0, via Wikimedia Commons

- o Genu varum/valgum: Standing so that patellae face anteriorly, and the medial aspect of knees and medial malleoli of both extremities are close together as much as possible.
    - Knees touch & Ankles don't touch: Genu valgum or Knock knee (9-10 cm distance between malleoli is considered excessive)

- Ankles touch & Knees don't touch: Genu varum or Bow knee (4 cm distance between knees is considered excessive)
- <u>Position of patella, tibia and feet:</u> Stand above the patient's knees & looking downwards along the tibial tuberosity and anterior tibial crest. The coronal plane of the knee is then compared with an imaginary line connecting the medial and lateral malleoli of the ankle.

Patella points	Feet points	Condition
Inward	Inward	Increased femoral anteversion
Outward	Outward	Femoral retroversion
Forward	Inward	Internal tibial torsion
Forward	Outward	External tibial torsion

Neutral feet	Axis of tibia falls on 2nd metatarsal
Hyperpronation or Overpronation	Axis of tibia falls medial to 2nd metatarsal
Hypersupination or Oversupination	Axis of tibia falls lateral to 2nd metatarsal

- <u>Fullness of peripatellar fossa:</u> Effusion
- <u>Patella size:</u>
    - Magna: Osteophytes
    - Breva: Hypoplasia

b. From lateral:

- Ask the patient to push the knees back and observe:
    - Flexion deformity of knee: Arthritic changes
    - Genu recurvatum or hyperextension: Generalized ligamentous laxity or Patella alta

c. From posterior:

- <u>Pelvic levelness:</u> For leg length inequality
- <u>Popliteal area:</u> Swellings (Baker's cyst, Semimembranosus bursa, Popliteal artery aneurysm, Lymphadenopathy, Soft tissue tumors)
- <u>Foot position:</u>

Neutral feet	Axis of feet/heel & Axis of leg is aligned		
Hyperpronation or Overpronation	Axis of feet/heel angles outward from Axis of leg	Common in people with flat foot	Leg shorten (LLD), Compensatory internal tibial torsion
Hypersupination or Oversupination	Axis of feet/heel angles inward from Axis of leg	Common in people with high arch foot	Leg lengthen (LLD)

d. **Walk (Gait):** Some important assessments and gaits in knee examination -

- <u>Foot progression angle (FPA):</u> Angle between direction of progression (walking) and long axis of foot (line between tip of heel & 2nd toe)

- - In-toeing (Negative FPA): Internal rotation of hip, Increased femoral anteversion, Internal tibial torsion
  - Out-toeing (Positive FPA): External rotation of hip, Femoral retroversion, External tibial torsion
- <u>Valgus thrust:</u> Increased valgus alignment on stance phase
  - Lateral compartment OA
  - Medial ligament laxity
  - Quadriceps weakness
- <u>Varus thrust:</u> Increased varus alignment on stance phase
  - Medial compartment OA
  - Lateral ligament laxity
  - Quadriceps weakness
- <u>Varus recurvatum:</u> Knee goes into recurvatum and varus on stance phase
  - Posterolateral laxity
- <u>Foot drop gait:</u> 20% of patients with these PLC injuries also have a common peroneal nerve palsy
- <u>Lateral perspective:</u> Recurvatum thrust gait, Stiff-knee gait

Sitting

1.   **Patient's position:** Sitting on 'W' position indicates excessive femoral anteversion

2.   **Patellar position (Seen from lateral):**

   - <u>Normal:</u> Anterior surface of patella must face the wall in front and patella must be centered in the soft tissue outline of knee (when seen from front)
   - <u>Patella alta:</u> More horizontal
   - <u>Patella baja:</u> More vertical

3.   **Vastus medialis obliquus (VMO)/Vastus lateralis relationship:**

   - With the knees held in 45° flexion:
     - <u>Normal:</u> distal 1/3 of vastus medialis has substantial muscle (from adductor tubercle insertion to upper medial patella)
     - <u>Dysplastic VMO:</u> hollow in normal location &/or apparent vastus lateralis hypertrophy

4. **Active extension and flexion of knee with legs handing over the couch:**

- <u>Crepitus:</u> tight deep lateral retinacular structures, cartilaginous or synovial lesions
- <u>Patellar tracking:</u> Normally straight or slight/smooth gradual, lateral concave "C"
  - **J sign:** Patella slips off laterally as knee approaches extension (sublux) & suddenly moves medially on flexion (engages the trochlea) <u>https://www.youtube.com/watch?v=3EegZYRyUns</u>
- <u>Quadriceps lag:</u> Muscle atrophy, pain, effusion, reflex inhibition (capsular stretching/increased intra-articular pressure) or loss of mechanical advantage
- <u>Ability to correct coronal malalignment in extension and flexion:</u>
  - Inability to correct a valgus deformity in both knee flexion and knee extension:

> a. Tight lateral collateral
> ligament, popliteus tendon
> or posterolateral capsule

- Inability to correct a valgus deformity in knee extension but not in flexion:
  - a. Tight iliotibial band

Supine

1. Best to observe swelling:
   - <u>Diffuse:</u> Effusion or synovial swelling
     - With red skin: Sepsis or gout
     - With muscular wasting: Severe and longstanding arthritis
   - <u>Localized:</u> Osteophytes, cysts, inflamed bursa
2. Patellar tracking: Asked for isometric quadriceps contraction → Positive if patella tracks more laterally than superiorly

Feel (Palpation)

Palpation is done mostly in 'supine' position. Remember the mnemonic **TEST Areas**.

Superficial

1.	Temperature (joint line, patella, suprapatellar pouch, femoral/tibial condyles, popliteal fossa, calf)
    * Increased temperature:
        o	Hemarthrosis
        o	Recent trauma or surgeries
        o	Arthritis (inflammatory, traumatic, septic)
        o	Loose body or impacted meniscus
        o	Fracture
        o	Metastases
        o	Osteitis deformans
        o	Ligamentous lesions
2.	Tenderness

Deep

a. With knee extended

1. <u>Test for effusion and Synovial swelling:</u> *Swelling without effusion = Synovial hypertrophy*

- <u>Juxta Patellar hollow:</u> Disappears in lesser angle of flexion if effusion
- <u>Cross fluctuation test (massive effusion):</u> One hand on suprapatellar pouch & other hand straddles front of joint below patella → feel for fluid impulse squeezing each hand alternately
- <u>Patellar tap test (moderate effusion; 50 ml):</u> Suprapatellar pouch emptied → tap patella back on femoral condyle
- <u>Wipe/Bulge test (small effusion; 15 ml):</u> Suprapatellar pouch emptied with one hand → Medial compartment emptied with upward stroke with another hand → Lateral aspect compressed downward with same hand → Ripple on flattened medial surface

- <u>Synovial swelling</u>: Best felt at the medial & lateral condyles of the femur, about 2 cm posterior to the medial and lateral edges of the patella (synovium lies almost superficially, covered only by skin and subcutaneous fat) by rolling the structures between fingertip & bone.
    - Normal: Only skin felt
    - Synovial thickening: Dense doughy structure can be felt

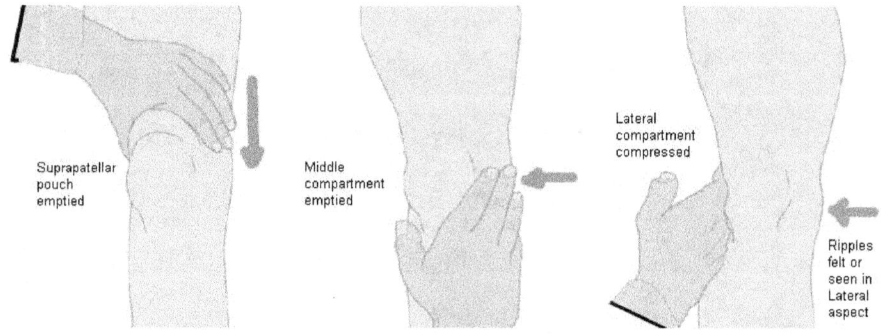

Patellar wipe/bulge test

2. <u>Patella and extensor apparatus:</u>

- Suparapatellar pouch
- Patella: Anterior surface → Edges → Posterior surface (facet; by pushing to one side then to another i.e. glide test)
- Parapatellar area

- Patellar tendon (tendinitis = Jumper's knee)

- Hoffa's fat pad (between patellar tendon and anterior capsule)

- Tibial tubercle (raised and tender in Osgood-Schlatter disease or Mortarmen's knee)

b. **Knees in 90° flexion:**

1. <u>Anterior:</u>

   - Patellar tendon:

     - Bassett's sign: Chronic patellar tendinosis

       a. Tenderness in proximal tendon is more in extension compared to flexion

       b. In flexion, the normal superficial fibers cover the damaged deep fibers, resulting in less pain on palpation

2. <u>Lateral:</u>

   - Lateral joint line (Tenderness = Most sensitive test for lateral meniscus tear)

   - Fibular head

- Lateral femoral condyle

- ITB and Gerdy's tubercle

3. <u>Medial:</u>

- Medial joint line (Tenderness = Most sensitive test for medial meniscus tear)

- Medial tibial condyle & Medial femoral condyle

- Pes anserinus (medially below joint line, just 2 cm from tibial tuberosity)

4. <u>Posterior (Poplitieal fossa):</u>

- Baker's cyst (below joint line)

- Semimebranous bursa (superior to joint line)

Move

Instruct the patient to perform active movements and then the examiner tries to observe for possible additional passive movements.

Describe the movements:

- Quantitatively: In degrees or distance

- Qualitatively: Smooth or Interrupted

- End-feel: Soft, Firm or Hard

Movement	Technique	Normal range	Comments
Flexion	Bend the knee & bring the heels towards buttock	0-150°	
	Heel to Buttock distance	Compared to other side	
	Passive flexion while palpating knee		To feel for crepitus: 1. Fine crepitus: May be normal in middle-aged individuals 2. Rough crepitus: Marked fragmentation of surface of articular cartilage 3. Hard creaking (of bone against bone):

			Complete erosion of articular cartilage
Extension	Straighten the knee pressing down on couch or Active straight leg raise	0°	
	Gap between knee & couch assessed by insertion of hand	No gap	
	Further, heels lifted by examiner (Passive extension)		Popliteal angle = Angle of fixed flexion deformity (FFD) Also look for hyperextension or recurvatum deformity

The popliteal angle is the angle subtended by the long axis of thigh and leg. Besides, flexion & extension internal rotation and external rotation of tibia can also be assessed with the knee in flexion while examiner stabilizes the femur & the position of tibial tubercle is assessed from neutral position (0-10°).

Beighton scale: for assessment of generalized ligamentous laxity

Measure

a. **Length:**

1. Apparent and true length; Femoral and tibial length

2. <u>Genu valgum:</u> Inter-malleolar distance

3. <u>Genu varum:</u> Distance between 2 knees

b. **Circumference:**

1. <u>Quadriceps wasting:</u> 15 cm from joint line (>2 cm = significant)

2. <u>Calf wasting:</u> 15 cm below joint line

3. <u>Effusion:</u> 5 cm above joint line

c. **Q-angle:**

- <u>Patient position:</u> Standing or Supine with Knee 30° flexed

- <u>Measurement:</u> Angle between –

    - Axis 1: ASIS to center of patella

    - Axis 2: Tibial tuberosity to center of patella

Neurovascular examination

- Motor
  - knee flexion – sciatic nerve
  - knee extension – femoral nerve
  - foot plantarflexion – tibial nerve
  - foot dorsiflexion – deep peroneal nerve
- Sensory
  - medial thigh – obturator nerve
  - anterior thigh – femoral nerve
  - posterolateral leg – sciatic nerve
  - dorsal foot – peroneal nerve
  - plantar foot – tibial nerve
- Pulses
  - popliteal
  - dorsal pedis
  - posterior tibial
- Reflexes
  - patellar (L4)
    - hypoactive/absent: L4 radiculopathy
    - hyperactive: UMN injury

Special tests

These tests are done with patients in supine position unless otherwise stated.

MCL & LCL

Varus/Valgus stress test: Examiner uses 1 hand as fulcrum and another hand to apply valgus (for MCL) or varus force (LCL) and opening of joint and endpoint (soft or hard) are noted –

1.   <u>30° knee flexion:</u> Relaxes secondary restraints → More specific for MCL/LCL

2.   <u>0° knee flexion (extension):</u> Additionally tests Cruciate ligaments and Capsule

- Increased laxity with valgus stress: MCL + Posteromedial capsule (Posterior-oblique ligament) &/or ACL injury

- Increased laxity with varus stress: LCL + PCL injury

Grade	Joint opening	End point	Significance
1	0-5 mm	Hard	Stretched ligament
2	5-10 mm	Hard	Partial ligament tear
3	>10 mm	Soft	Complete ligament tear

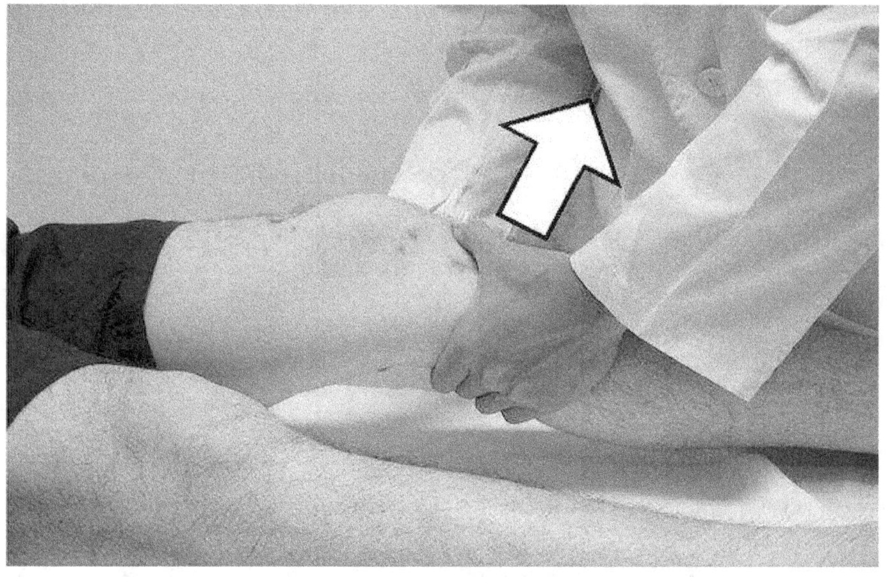

Lachmann test

Mak-Ham Lam, Daniel TP Fong, Patrick SH Yung, Eric PY Ho, Wood-Yee Chan and Kai-Ming Chan, CC BY-SA 2.0, via Wikimedia Commons

ACL & PCL

1. **Identify posterior sag or Godfrey sign:** With hip flexed 45° and knee flexed 90°, observe from side.

   - <u>Normal:</u> Medial tibial plateau extends about 5-10 mm anteriorly beyond the femoral condyle
   - <u>Positive posterior sag sign (PCL dysfunction):</u> Loss of the step-off between medial tibial plateau and femoral condyle on inspection and palpation
     - Grade I: 5 mm difference in posterior translation from normal side
     - Grade II: Tibia and femoral condyles are flush
     - Grade III: Tibia is posterior to femoral condyles

2. **Quadriceps active test (if posterior sag sign in positive):** With hip & knee is drawer position with foot fixed, patient is asked to extend the knee. If there is posterior sag, quadriceps will pull the tibia forward (correction of posterior sag).

3. **Lachman's test (most sensitive test for ACL):**

- Grasp the distal femur with one hand holding the femur still while flexing the knee 20-30° and displace the tibia anteriorly with another hand (thumb over anterior joint line)
- Tests posterolateral (PL) band of ACL as it is the primary restraint at 20° of flexion
- Isolates ACL by relaxing capsule and other secondary restraints, the collaterals
- With acute injuries patients are less apprehensive with 30° knee flexion compared to 90°
- Avoids "door-stopper" effect of meniscus
- <u>Grading</u>:
    - A = firm endpoint; B = no firm endpoint
    - Grade 1: <5 mm translation
    - Grade 2 A/B: 5-10 mm translation
    - Grade 3 A/B: >10 mm translation

4. **Anterior and posterior drawer test:**

- Posterior sag must be corrected first
- Palpate the hamstrings behind the knee to confirm if it is relaxed
- Knees are flexed to 90° and feet are fixed in neutral position on couch by sitting on the

patient's feet, the tibia is grasped with both thumbs on tibial tubercle and pulled forwards (anterior drawer test) and pushed backwards (posterior drawer test) from neutral position

- <u>Grading for posterior drawer test:</u>

Grade	Posterior translation	Tibial position with posterior drawer
0	<5 mm	Normal knee
1+	5-10 mm	Tibial plateau still remains anterior to femoral condyles
2+	10-15 mm	Tibial plateau even with femoral condyles
3+	>15 mm	Tibial plateau posterior to femoral condyles

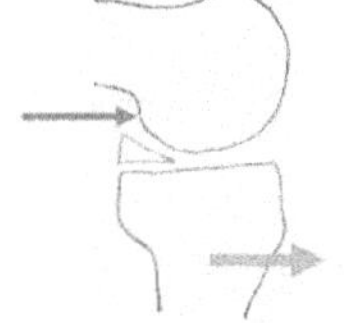

90º Flexion

Anterior drawer test

Less sensitive

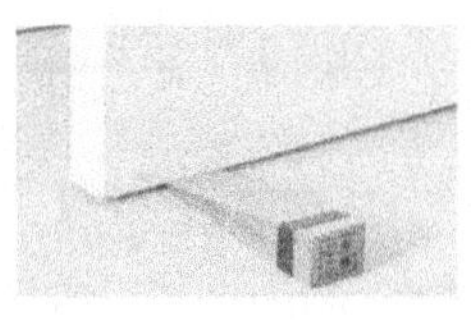

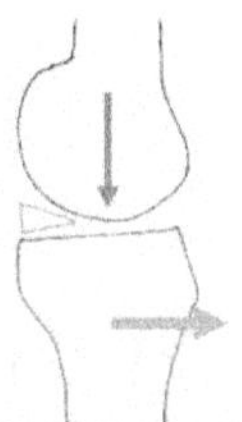

0-20 º Flexion

Lachman test

More sensitive

"Door stop effect"

5. **Lelli's (Lever) test:**

- A clenched fist (fulcrum) is placed beneath the proximal calf just distal to tibial tuberosity and gentle downwards pressure is applied over quadriceps tendon and the examiner looks to see if the heel 'lifts off' the bed.
    - Negative test (ACL intact): Heel lifts off the bed
    - Positive test (ACL injured): Ruptured ACL is not able to counteract the downward force on the foot and the foot remains on the examination table
- Lever Sign test was more sensitive to correctly diagnose both acute and partial tears of the ACL, regardless of the elapsed time from injury, compared with other common manual tests

Rotatory Instabilities

1. **Posterolateral rotatory instability:** Posterolateral corner (PLC) comprises LCL, popliteus tendon, posterolateral ligament complex, fabellofibular ligament.

- <u>External rotation recurvatum test:</u> Knees extended → Grab toes of both feet and lift the feet off the table
  - Positive: Abnormal knee falls into recurvatum and varus, tibia externally rotated compared to normal knee
- <u>Modified posterolateral drawer test:</u> Posterior drawer test with feet in maximum in external rotation
  - Positive: External rotation of tibia (tibial tubercle in relation to distal femur)
    - Indicative of grade III posterolateral corner (PLC) injury
- <u>Dial or Loomer test:</u> Patient is positioned Prone → Thigh foot angle is measured at 30° and 90° flexion → >10 degree difference = positive
  - Positive at 30° and 90° = combined instability (PCL + PLC)
  - Positive at 30° only = Isolated PLC injury
- <u>Reverse pivot test (Jakob):</u> Foot is externally rotated with right hand → Left hand is placed on proximal tibia → Knee is flexed to to 70° (Tibia subluxes posterolaterally) → Knee is then

extended to 20° (Reduction as ITB becomes extensor at this position)

- Suggestive of combined PLC and PCL injury

- Modified Hughston Classification:

Grade	I (Mild)	II (Mod.)	III (Sev.)
Varus stress – lateral opening at 30° knee flexion	0-5 mm	6-10 mm	>10 mm
Dial test – rotational instability	0-5°	6-10°	>10°

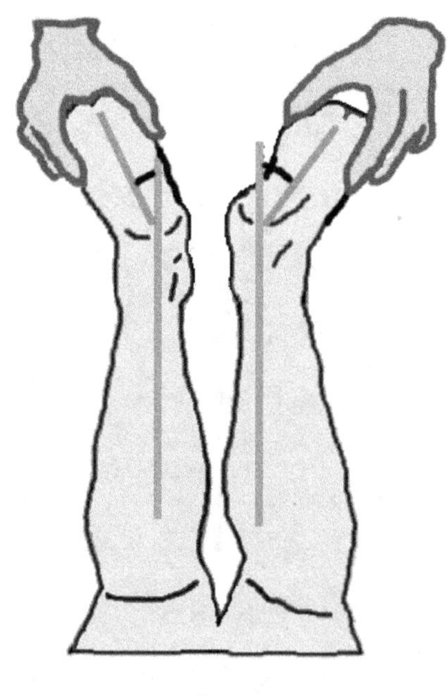

Dial test

2. **Anterolateral and Anteromedial rotatory instability:**

- <u>Pivot shift test (ALRI):</u> Foot internally rotated on extended knee → Valgus stress → At 30° flexion (sublux position) → Flex to >40° (Reduction by ITB) or Extend (Reduction)
    - The knee to be tested should be fully extended and the hip flexed to approximately 30°. One of the examiner's hands holds the heel of the foot of the leg to be tested in internal rotation. Examiner's other hand is on the lateral aspect of the proximal tibia
    - Slowly flex the knee while putting a moderate valgus and internal rotation force
    - Positive: Proximal tibia subluxes anteriorly on distal femur at about 30° of flexion & clunk back into place while returning the knee to extension and flexion past approximately 40° (iliotibial band will act as flexor)
        - Indicates ACL + ALL (Anterolateral ligament) injury

- With positive test, ALL reconstruction or Anterolateral tenodesis is recommended
- With partial ACL tears:
  - Pivot shift negative: Conservative treatment may be tried
  - Pivot shift positive: ACL reconstruction recommended

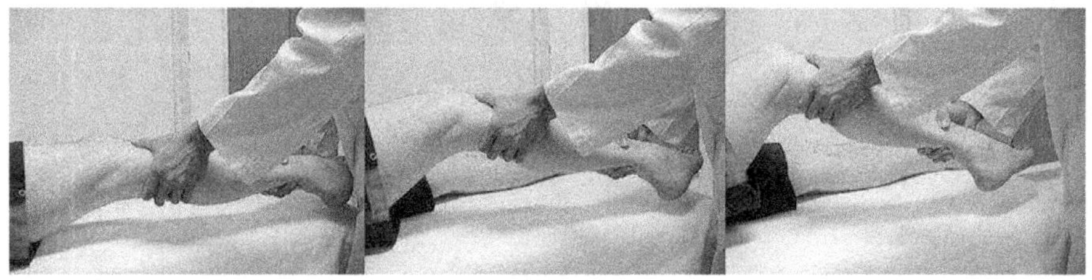

Pivot shift test: Internal rotation & valgus stress on extended knee which is slowly flexed

Mak-Ham Lam, Daniel TP Fong, Patrick SH Yung, Eric PY Ho, Wood-Yee Chan and Kai-Ming Chan, CC BY-SA 2.0, via Wikimedia Commons

- **Slocum test:** Anterior drawer test in maximal internal or external rotation of foot

- Subluxation of anteromedial tibial plateau on external rotation: Anteromedial rotatory instability (AMRI)
  - Injured structures: Posteromedial capsule (PMC) + MCL
- Subluxation of anterolateral tibial plateau on internal rotation: Anterolateral rotatory instability (ALRI)
  - Injured structures: ACL + LCL &/or Arcuate ligament

Meniscus

1. **McMurray's test:** Stay on side of patient → Maximally flex hip and knee → Grasp foot (thumb lateral and other fingers inside) → Thumb of other hand against lateral aspect knee → External rotation (medial meniscus) or Internal rotation (lateral meniscus), i.e. loose meniscus trapping position → Extend knee (Reduction) → Audible click or palpable click/thud

- Repeated several times with application of varus/valgus stress

- Most specific for tear of posterior horn of meniscus medial meniscus becomes more anterior in extension and external rotation.

Mnemonic: *The heel points towards the meniscus tested.*

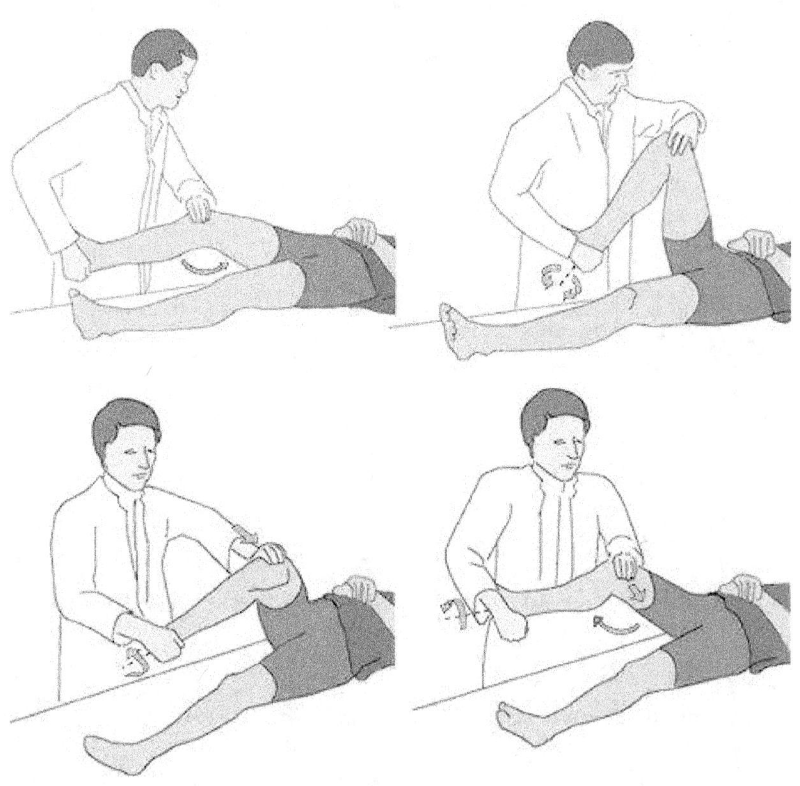

Illustration of mcmurray test for meniscus tear – McMurrays Test – WikiSM (Sports Medicine Wiki)

2. **Apley's grind test:** Patient is placed prone → Flex the knee to 90° → Stabilize thigh with examiner's knee → Positive on compression with rotation (meniscus pathology) → Positive on distraction with rotation (collateral ligament pathology)

- Internal rotation for Lateral meniscus and LCL
- External rotation of Medial meniscus and MCL

3. **Thessaly test:** One knee flexed to 20° on single leg stance (standing) → Hold the patient's hands to prevent overbalancing → Twist his/her body to one then other side for 3 times (stand on unaffected leg as a trial, then on affected leg)

- <u>Positive:</u> Medial/Lateral joint line pain/locking/clicking
- Most accurate for meniscal pathology

4. **Other tests:**

- <u>Squat test:</u> Reproduces mechanical pain on affected knee
- <u>Duck walk (Childress test):</u> Joint line pain

- <u>Steinmann test:</u> Patient seated & with knee hanging loose over the edge of the table- knee flexed at least 90 degrees, foot grasped & tibia is sharply rotated into internal rotation then external rotation- a meniscal lesion is demonstrated by pain at the appropriate joint line
- <u>Figure of 4 test:</u> The affected leg is positioned in figure of 4 → examiner pushes involved knee towards the bed
  - Pain over lateral joint line: Popliteomeniscal tear (lateral meniscus instability)
  - Pain over medial joint line (payr sign): Posterior horn of medial meniscus injury

Patellofemoral

1. **Osmond-Clarke's test:** Hand over suprapatellar pouch with gentle pressure on superior pole of patella → Ask to contract quadriceps or straight leg raise → Pain in patellofemoral joint (chondromalacia/arthritis)

https://epomedicine.com/clinical-medicine/clarkes-test/

2. **Patellar glide test (Sage test):** Flex the knee to $30^{\circ} \rightarrow$ Move patella maximally medially and laterally

- <u><1 quadrant (of patellar width) medial glide:</u> Lateral retinacular tightness

- <u>>3 quadrant lateral glide:</u> Medial retinacular laxity

  - Also look for apprehension: In cases of instability, patella tends to slip over the lateral condyle of the femur & the patient suddenly contracts the quadriceps muscle and draws the patella back.

3. **Patellar tilt or eversion test:** Knee straight and relaxed $\rightarrow$ Put both the thumbs on lateral border of patella and both the index fingers on the medial border of patella $\rightarrow$ Push the patella medially with thumbs & evert the medial surface using index fingers (Medial patellar eversion test) or Push the patella laterally with index fingers & evert the lateral surface using thumbs (Lateral patellar eversion test)

- <u>Patella cannot be everted beyond horizontal:</u> Medial or Lateral patellar retinaculum tightness

- Excessive medial patellar eversion compared to opposite: MPFL (Medial patellofemoral ligament) disruption

4. **Moving patellar apprehension test:** Knee straight and relaxed (at the edge of bed) → Patella is pushed laterally with one hand → Knee is taken into passive flexion with another hand

   - Positive: Patient resists further flexion out of apprehension and indicates lateral patellar instability

5. **Relocation test for medial patellar instability:** Knee straight and relaxed → Patella is pushed medially with one hand (subluxates) → Knee is taken into passive flexion with another hand while pressure on patella is released

   - Positive: Patient experiences pain, apprehension or reproduction of symptoms as the patella relocates (Extensor mechanism pulls the patella laterally with tension on flexion)

6.   **Rotational profile (Prone examination):**

- <u>Tibial torsion (Thigh foot angle):</u>
  - Patient lies prone with knee flexed to 90º and the ankle is positioned in neutral dorsiflexion. Consider:
    - A line passing along the long axis of the thigh
    - A line passing along the long axis of the foot
  - The angle between the two lines is the thigh-foot angle, which is a measure of tibial version (internal tibial version if foot pointing inwards, external tibial version if foot pointing outwards). Normal value in adults is about 10-15º of external rotation.
- <u>Femoral anteversion:</u>
  <u>https://epomedicine.com/clinical-medicine/femoral-anteversion-craigs-test/</u>

__Alternative method for measuring tibial torsion:__
The transmalleolar axis can be used in the sitting position by comparing the transcondylar axis of the tibia with the bimalleolar axis, which is usually about 20º of external rotation.

Other Special Tests

1. **Hoffa's test:** Hip and Knee flexed 45° → Examiner presses with both thumbs on either side of patellar tendon just below inferior pole of patella → Patient is asked to extend the knee actively

- ○ <u>Positive:</u> Pain at the level of patellar tendon due to impingement of infrapatellar fat pad

2. **Medial Patellar Plica (MPP) test:** Knee extended → Examiner presses inferomedial part of patellofemoral joint (compressing the medial plica between the medial femoral condyle & patella) → Knee is flexed to 90°

- ○ <u>Positive:</u> Pain with knee extension but minimal or no pain on knee flexion

3. **Wilson's test (for Osteochondritis Dissecans):** Patient sitting on edge of table with legs hanging → Axial compression at knee by pushing proximally → The knee is taken into passive extension

- <u>Positive:</u> Pain at approximately 30° flexion with tibia in internal rotation but no pain or discomfort with external rotation of tibia
    - Internal rotation causes impingement of the tibial eminence on the OCD lesion of the medial femoral condyle which causes the pain
- Absent in most patients with medial femoral condyle OCD
- If present, it may signify resolution of the lesion when the test becomes negative

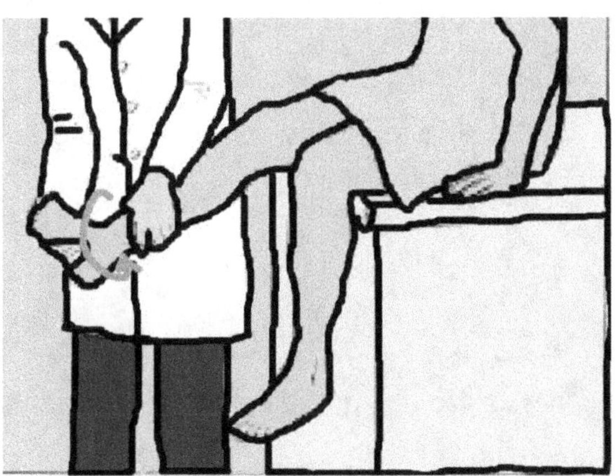

Wilson's test for medial femoral condyle OCD (Osteochondritis Dissecans)

Completion

Spine, Hip, SIJ examination

The back, sacroiliac joint, and hip commonly refer pain to the knee.

- The L5 root and sacroiliac joint refer pain down the back of the leg to the popliteal space.
- The S1 root, the trochanteric bursa, and the femur refer pain down the outer thigh to the lateral area of the knee.
- The hip joint and the femur refer pain down the front of the thigh to the anterior knee.

Referred pain is suggested whenever the patient's pain is not well localized, the knee exam is free of local tenderness or inflammatory changes, and the flexion and extension of the knee are normal.

CHAPTER 9

Cervical Spine Examination

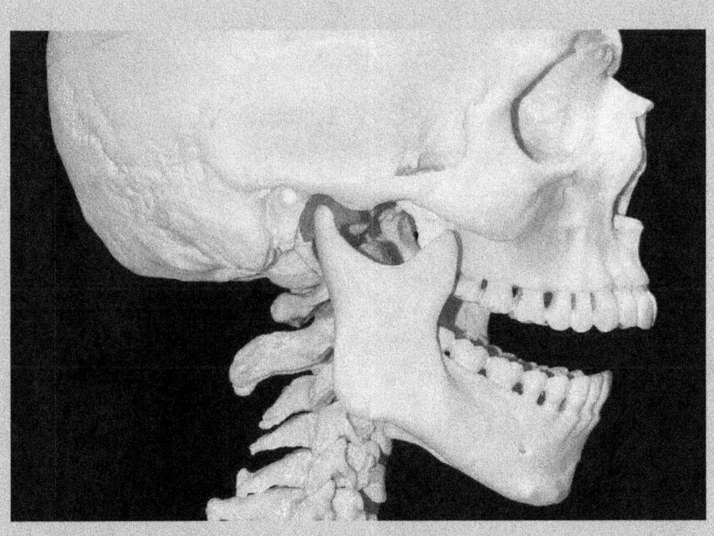

Cervical Spine Examination

The cervical spine examination is crucial for accurate diagnosis, early intervention, prevention of chronic pain, reduced risk of complications, integration with other examinations & identification of red flags.

Exposure

Ask the patient to remove enough clothing for you to see the neck and upper thorax.

Look

Remember the mnemonic **SEADS GO**. Inspection is done in Standing position.

The head should be held erect, centered over the pelvis and perpendicular to the floor, while the patient maintains a horizontal gaze.

a. Anterior view:

- Horizontal head shift: Disc protrusion
- Slight head tilt: Normal or Cervical joint dysfunction

b. Lateral view: Chin tip should be in line with manubrium

- Head forward to the line: Excessive lordosis (Shortened neck extensors)
- Head backward to the line: Flattened lordosis (Shortened neck flexors)

c. Posterior view:

- Posterior hairline
- Appearance of no neck (Sprengel's deformity)
- Upper trapezius and sternocleidomastoid prominence

Feel

Remember the mnemonic **TEST Areas**.

Superficial

- Temperature
- Tenderness

Deep

a. Anterior: In sitting or supine position

- <u>Bone & Cartilages:</u>
    - Hyoid (C3)
    - Thyroid cartilage (C4-C5) and thyroid gland
    - Cricoid (C6)
    - Carotid tubercle of C6 (found by moving laterally from cricoid ring)
    - Trachea (any deviation from midline or abnormal findings)
- <u>Soft tissues:</u>
    - Carotid pulse (one at a time; never both sides at the same time)
    - Supraclavicular fossa (lymph nodes, cervical rib or tumors)

- Sternocleidomastoid & mastoid process (lymph nodes, prominence in torticollis)
- Parotid gland

b. Posterior: In sitting or prone position

- <u>Bone:</u>
  - Posterior occipital area (tenderness, abnormal masses, bony protuberance)
  - C2-T1 spinous process (pain/tenderness, swelling of paraspinal muscles)
  - Facet joints – lateral to spinous process (tenderness)
- <u>Soft tissues:</u>
  - Trapezius (tenderness in whiplash flexion injuries or shoulder disorders)
  - Greater occipital nerve (palpable/hyperaesthetic in whiplash injuries)
  - Superior nuchal ligament (inion to C7 spinous process)
    - Generalized tenderness: Whiplash injury

- Localized tenderness: Cervical spondylotic disease

Move

Assess active movements 1st. If active movements are reduced, gently perform passive movements and record:

- Quantitative: Range of motion
- Qualitative: Smooth or Interrupted
- End-feel
- Pain or Paresthesia

a. Forward flexion: Ask the patient to put his chin on the chest

- <u>Normal:</u> 0-80° (Chin touches chest)
- Record limitations in degrees or distance between chin to chest

b. Extension: Ask the patient to look upwards at ceiling as far back as possible

- Normal: 0-50° (in full extension – occipitomental line forms 45° with horizontal)

c. Lateral flexion or bending: Ask the patient to put his ear on the shoulder without shrugging

- Normal: 0-45° (Ear touches shoulder)

d. Rotation: Ask the patient to look over his/her shoulder

- Normal: 0-80°

Screen

a. Gait:

- Slow, wide-based, unsteady gait: Cervical myelopathy

b. Tandem gait (Heel to toe):

- Unable to walk on a straight line: Cerebellar disorder

c. Romberg test:

- Positive Romberg test: Sensory ataxia

Neurologic Examination

For motor testing:

- Joint should be in resting position before testing
- Contraction must be held atleast 5 seconds
- Use mMRC scale for grading motor function (1-5)

For sensory testing:

- Grade sensory findings as:
    - 0 – absent sensation
    - 1 – altered sensation
    - 2 – normal sensation
- Score major sensory types in all patients
    - pain (sharp object like paper clip)
    - light touch (stroke lightly with finger)
- Score minor sensory types for focused exam
    - vibration (focused exam)

- temperature (focused exam)
- two-point discrimination (focused exam)

Root	Primary motion	Tested muscles	Sensory	Reflex
C2-C4	Shrugging of shoulders	Trapezius Levator scapulae Rhomboids	Back of skull & neck	
C5	Shoulder abduction Elbow flexion (in supination)	Deltoid Biceps	Lateral arm below deltoid	Biceps
C6	Elbow flexion (in neutral) Wrist extension	Brachioradialis ECRL	Thumb & radial hand or forearm	Brachio-radialis
C7	Elbow extension Wrist flexion	Triceps FCR	Middle finger	Triceps
C8	Finger flexion Hand grip Thumb extension	FDS	Little finger	
T1	Finger abduction	Interossei muscles	Medial elbow	

Special tests

Provocative maneuvers

1. **Spurling test or Foraminal compression test:** Stand behind the seated patient, support his/her shoulder with one hand & move the head into a slight rotation (to opposite side) and side bend to one side, while at the same time extending the patient's neck with another hand. Now add a brief axial compression to the head.

- <u>Positive:</u> Radiating pain (indicates root compression)
- <u>Abduction relief sign:</u> If the test is positive, abduct the arm overhead –
    - Pain relieved: Root compression
    - Pain increased: Increased pressure on interscalene triangle

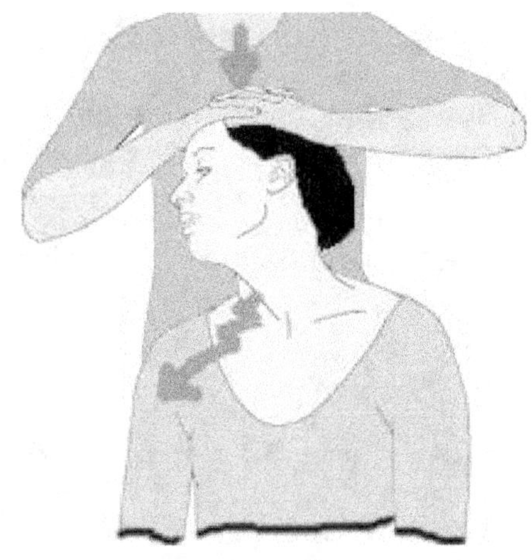

Spurling's test

2. **Axial separation or Cervical distraction test:** Examiner places one hand on chin and another on occiput of the seated patient and applies axial traction.

- ○ <u>Symptom reduction:</u> Neck traction might be beneficial

3. **Lhermitte's test or Phenomenon:** Ask the patient to flex the head forward, and determine if symptoms occur in a shooting fashion down the arms and/or legs.

- ○ <u>Positive:</u> Anterior compressive lesions (cervical myelopathy)

4. **Valsalva test:** Instruct the patient to hold the breath and bear down, as when lifting weights improperly or straining to empty the bowels. If this action produces or increases preexisting pain or other symptomatology, the test is positive.

- ○ <u>Positive (note the dermatome):</u> Space occupying lesions (herniated discs or tumors)

Tests for Vertebrobasilar Syndrome

1. **DeKleyn test (Vertebral artery test):** Have the patient rest in a supine position with the head over the edge of the exam table. Instruct the patient to hyperextend & rotate head for 15-30 seconds. Repeat on the opposite side.

- <u>Positive:</u> Vertigo, dizziness, visual blurring, nystagmus, nausea, faintness

If the patient complains of dizziness, vestibular dysfunction must be ruled out before considering vertebrobasilar syndrome.

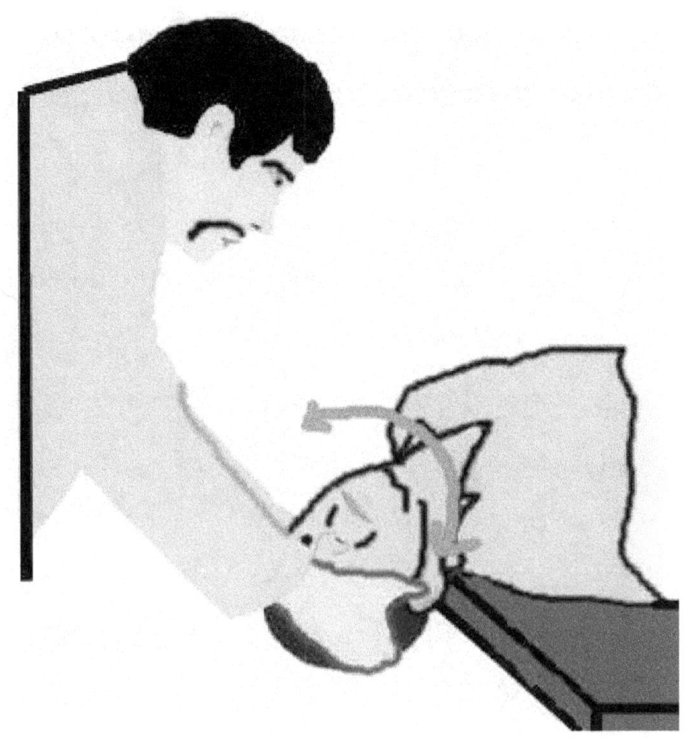

DeKleyn's test

2. **Hautant's test**: Patient stands or seats with eyes closed & both arms flexed forwards with palms up (supinated). Instruct the patient to extend the neck & rotate his head on each side which is held for 30 seconds.

- <u>Positive:</u> Loss of balance, Dropping of arms or Pronator drift (Vertebrobasilar insufficiency)

3. **Vertebral Artery Motion Test:** Stand in front of the standing patient & stabilize his/her shoulders. Instruct the patient to rapidly rotate the head from side to side for 10 seconds or until symptoms are reproduced. If the exam produces symptoms, check to see if the pupils are symmetric. Asymmetric
pupils after the vertebral artery motion test may indicate reduced blood flow through one of
the vertebral arteries.

Tests for Thoracic Outlet Syndrome

1. **Adson's test:** Have the patient seated and feel his/her radial pulse with arm slightly abducted & externally rotated with elbow in extension. Ask the patient to inhale deep breath & hold while he/she extends the neck & rotates the head towards the examined side (chin up & towards examined side).

- <u>Positive:</u> Decrease or absence of radial pulse (Subclavian artery compression at Thoracic outlet)
  - Cervical rib

○ Tightened scalene muscles (anticus & medius)

2. **Roos test or Elevated Arm Stress Test (EAST):** Have the patient seated with shoulders abducted to 90° in external rotation & elbows flexed to 90° & ask the patient to open & clench fist for 3 minutes.

● <u>Positive:</u> Inability to complete test, patient drops arm or reproduction of neurologic symptoms

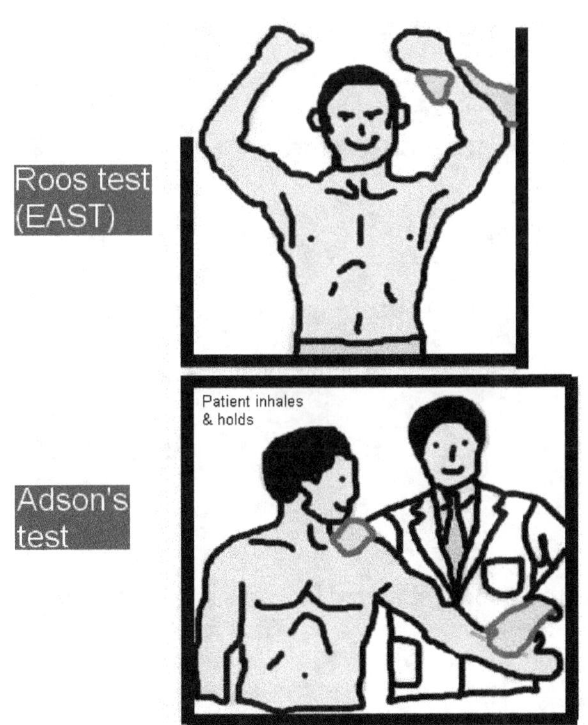

3. **Hyperabduction (Wright) test:** Have the patient seated and palpate his/her radial pulse while the shoulder is passively taken into hyperabduction.

- <u>Positive:</u> Decreased radial pulse or reproduction of symptoms (Pectoralis minor syndrome)
    - Components of neurovascular bundle are pulled around pectoralis minor tendon, the coracoid process & head of humerus

4. **Costoclavicular test (Military brace or Eden's test):** Have the patient seated while the examiner palpates the radial pulse on wrist while passively drawing the arm inferiorly and posteriorly.

- <u>Positive:</u> Decreased radial pulse or reproduction of symptoms (Costoclavicular syndrome)

Tests for Cervical Myelopathy

1. **Hoffmann's test:** Flick the nail of the middle finger

- Positive: Muscles of the hand and thumb flex

  (UMN lesion above T1)

  https://youtu.be/cDtBS1fnMXg

2. **Finger escape or Wartenberg's sign:** Ask the patient to extend and adduct their fingers and maintain that position for up to a minute.

- Positive: Small finger drifts into abduction (overpowered radial nerve innervated EDM and weak ulnar nerve innervated palmar interossei)
  - Ulnar nerve palsies
  - Cervical myelopathy

3. **Grip and release test:** Patient is asked to rapidly repeat the clenching of fist and releasing it.

- Positive: <20 times in 10 seconds
- Can improve after the management of disease

Findings and other tests in cervical myelopathy:

Upper extremity	Lower extremity	Additional
Decreased hand dexterity	Impairment of gait and/or falls	Lhermitte's phenomenon
Lower motor neuron signs (muscle weakness, atrophy, fasciculation, hyporeflexia, hypotonia)	Upper motor neuron signs (weakness, hyperreflexia, hypertonia)	Incontinence
Change in pain, temperature, proprioception, dermatomal sensation	Change in pain, temperature, proprioception, dermatomal sensation	Neck pain
Motor deficits	Motor deficits	
Thenar atrophy	Babinski reflex	
Hoffman sign	Romberg test	
Inverted radial reflex	Sustained foot clonus	
Finger escape sign		
Grip and release test		
Hyperactive pectoralis reflex		

Completion

1. **Waddel's signs for Non-organic causes (in chronic neck pain):**
   a. Superficial tenderness with light touch or pinching
   b. Non-anatomical tenderness
   c. Sensory loss that is not dermatomal, motor loss in a non-anatomical pattern, strictly midline to lateral symptoms
   d. Overreaction during the examination
2. Carotid artery Auscultation (for bruit)
3. Examination of lower cranial nerves (IX, XI, and XIII)
4. Oropharyngeal examination

CHAPTER 10

Shoulder Examination

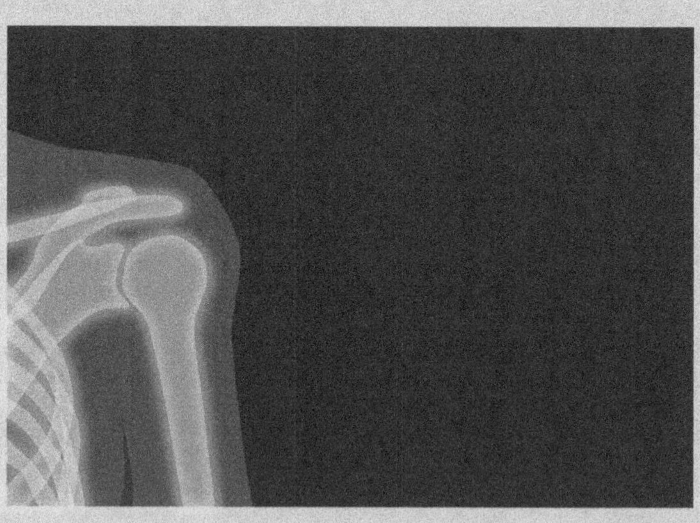

Shoulder Examination

Examination of the shoulder is complex due to unique biomechanical and structural changes, multiple joint articulations, multiple pain patterns, and the potential of injury to intra-articular & extra-articular structures. Many shoulder examination tests thought to be unique to a single structure, joint, or condition can be positive in multiple conditions.

Exposure

Patients must be undressed to the waist and any garments worn should leave the scapulae visible.

Look

Overall (General)

- Comfortable at rest or in discomfort?

- Ask the patient to stand and walk a few steps – note overall posture, balance and mobility of lower and upper extremities.
- Look for SEADS from front, side and back sequentially.

From front

- ACJ or SCJ prominence: Degenerative or Traumatic (subluxation)
- Deformity of clavicle: Malunion
- Abduction + External rotation: Anterior shoulder dislocation or Pyogenic infections
- Adduction + Internal rotation: Posterior shoulder dislocation
- "Squared off" shoulder: Deltoid wasting
- "Pop-eye sign" (a dip between biceps and deltoid): Ruptured long head of biceps
- Loss of anterior axillary fold: Ruptured pectoralis major
- Deltopectoral groove incisions: Previous shoulder surgery

From side

- Look for deltoid wasting

From back

- Trapezius atrophy: Disuse or spinal accessory nerve lesion
- Small and high scapula: Sprengel's shoulder or Klippel-Feil syndrome (also webbed neck)
- Hollowing of supraspinous or infraspinous fossa: Chronic tears of supraspinatus or infraspinatus respectively or a suprascapular nerve lesion
- Prominence of shoulder blade (scapular winging): Ipsilateral serratus anterior muscle weakness (usually secondary to long thoracic nerve injury)
- Scoliosis and Kyphosis: Exaggerated kyphosis - risk for dynamic impingement syndrome
- "Soft spot" (1 cm medial & 2 cm inferior to posterolateral angle of acromion): Fullness indicates swelling

Feel

Superficial

- Temperature: Rises in inflammation & infection
- Tenderness

Deep

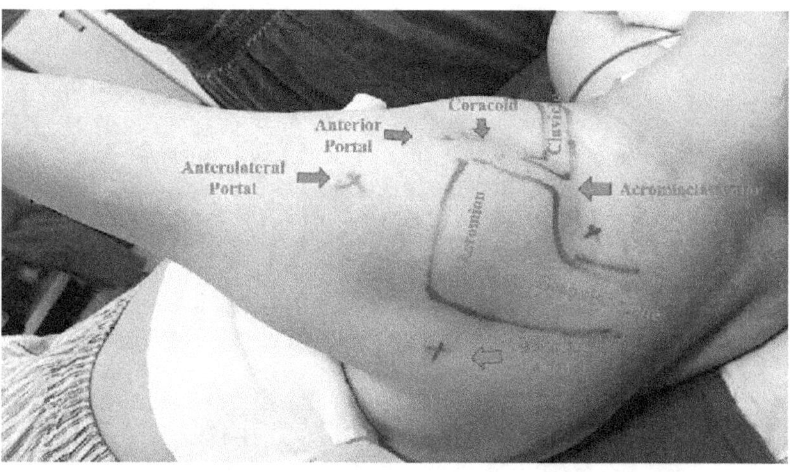

Zhou, Min & Zhou, Chuanhai & Zhang, Jin-Ming & Yi, Long & Guo, Jiang & Hou, Jing-Yi & Yang, Rui. (2022). The Lark Loop Used for Proximal Biceps Tenodesis: An All-Arthroscopic Technique. Arthroscopy Techniques. 11. 10.1016/j.eats.2022.02.031. [CC-BY 4.0]

From front:

- <u>SCJ:</u> Tenderness in –
    - Dislocations
    - Infections (TB)
    - Radionecrosis (post-breast cancer treatment)
- <u>Clavicle:</u> Palpate for tenderness and length of clavicle
- <u>ACJ:</u>
    - Vertical instability: Coraco-clavicular ligament disruption
    - Horizontal instability: Acromio-clavicular ligament disruption
- <u>Antero-lateral subacromial margins:</u> Tenderness during arc of shoulder abduction –
    - Rotator cuff tear, tendinitis or impingement
    - Bursitis
- <u>Anterior and posterior shoulder joint lines:</u> Diffuse tenderness –
    - Calcific supraspinatus tendinitis
    - Infection (marked tenderness in gonococcal infections)

- <u>Coracoid:</u>
    - Coracoid tenderness:
        - Pectoralis minor tendinopathy or tear
        - Conjoined tendon tendinopathy
        - Adhesive capsulitis (when associated with shoulder stiffness)
        - Fractures
        - Tumors
    - Tenderness inferior to coracoid: Coracoid impingement
- <u>Bicipital groove</u> (1 inch down from anterolateral tip of acromion in neutral rotation): Tenderness indicates bicipital tendinitis
- <u>Axilla:</u>
    - Humeral head: Exostoses of proximal humerus may be palpable
    - Enlarged lymph nodes

From side:

- <u>Deltoid bulk</u>
- <u>Step deformity:</u> Inferior subluxation of shoulder

From back:

- <u>Cervical spine and paraspinal muscles:</u> Trapezial cervical strain & cervical radiculopathy account for 15% of shoulder pain cases
- "<u>Soft spot</u>" for swelling
- <u>Subscapular bursa</u> (rib closest to supero-medial angle of scapula with the arm fully abducted such that the hand is placed on the contralateral shoulder): Tenderness is the hallmark of subscapular bursitis

Move

Cervical spine

- Flexion, extension, rotation, lateral flexion
- Patients whose pain is aggravated solely by neck rotation or lateral flexion rather than shoulder movement usually have an isolated cervical strain or radiculopathy.

Shoulder

Instruct the patient to perform bilateral active motion simultaneously and demonstrate the patient using own arms. Look for additional passive motion over patient-performed active motion. Describe motions under 2 headings:

- <u>Quantitative:</u> Degrees or how far the extended thumb can reach (in case of internal rotation)
  - Total motion (Glenohumeral + Scapulothoracic)
  - Individual movements: Examiner stabilizes the scapula with hand –
    - ROM before scapular motion starts: Glenohumeral ROM
    - ROM after scapular motion starts: Scapulothoracic ROM
- <u>Qualitative:</u> Smooth or Interrupted

a. From front:

- Abduction

- Adduction in extension

- Internal rotation in extension (reach chest)

- External rotation in extension

- Elevation & depression

b. From side:

- Forward flexion/elevation

- Extension

- Internal rotation in abduction

- External rotation in abduction

c. From above:

- Adduction in flexion (cross chest adduction)

d. From back:

- Internal rotation in extension (reach opposite scapula or small of back)

- Scapular protraction and retraction

Move	Maneuver	Range	Comments
Abduction	Ask the patient to raise arms sideways Normal shoulder – arm can touch the ear with only slight tilting of head	0-170°	Scapular rotation coupled with external rotation of the arm (proximal humerus) to take the greater tuberosity out of the subacromial space allows a full abduction normally. Initiation difficulty: Major rotator cuff tear Pain during 60-120° (painful arc): Subacromial impingement Pain after 120° abduction: Rotator cuff impingement in ACJ or coraco-acromial ligament, ACJ osteoarthritis Patient can hold the arm in vertical

			position: Deltoid & axillary nerve are likely intact
			Patient suddenly drops the arm when brining from vertical position to 90° abduction: Major rotator cuff tear
			If both active & passive ROM restricted (fix the inferior angle of scapula with 1 hand & try to abduct arm with another hand): Absence of movement (fixed glenohumeral joint; only scapulohumeral movements present)
Adduction in extension	Place one hand on shoulder & swing the arm, flexed at the	0-50°	

	elbow across the chest		
Forward flexion (observe from side)	Ask the patient to swing the arm forwards & lift it above his head	0-165°	
Backward extension (observe from side)	Ask the patient to swing the arm backwards & observe from the side	0-60°	
Horizontal flexion & adduction (observe from top)	Arm is moved forwards from a position of 90° abduction (cross chest adduction)	0-140°	Pain: ACJ osteoarthritis
Internal rotation in extension	Ask the patient to place the hand behind opposite scapula (Apley scratch test)	Quantify how high the extended thumb reaches: a. Lower angle of	Restricted: Frozen shoulder

	Ask the patient to move the hand to the chest	scapula (normal) b. "Small" of back (functional) 70°	
External rotation in extension	Ask the patient to stick the elbow to the sides with elbow flexed 90° and move the hands laterally	70°	Increased: Subscapularis tear Restricted: Teres minor tear/dysfunction
Internal rotation in 90° abduction	With elbow flexed to 90° and ask the patient to lower the forearm from horizontal plane	70°	

| External rotation in 90° abduction | Ask the patient to place both hands behind the head with elbows in horizontal plane

With elbow flexed to 90° & forearm parallel to ground, ask the patient to raise the hand | 100° | Restriction: Frozen shoulder or Glenohumeral arthritis |
| Shoulder elevation & depression | Use goniometer – 1 arm centered over jugular notch & another arm on acromion | 37° & 8° respectively | Elevation: Tests trapezius function

Restricted elevation & depression: Condition involving scapulothoracic motion |

Scapular protraction & retraction	Ask the patient to bring forward scapulae in 'hunched position' (protraction) & to pull back the shoulders in 'attention position' (retraction)		Alternation protraction & retraction may elicit 'snapping scapula' syndrome

Measure (Not usually performed)

- Apparent length: C7 to radial styloid
  - Causes of apparent LLD of upper limbs (compensatory tilt of shoulders):
    - Angular deformities at shoulder and elbow or bone shaft
    - Problems in neck (neck spasm/torticollis)
    - Spine (scoliosis)
    - Tilt of pelvis (LLD of lower limbs)
- Arm length: Angle of acromion to lateral epicondyle

- Mid-arm circumference: At the midpoint of acromion and olecranon

Neurovascular examination

- <u>Assess C4-T1:</u> dermatomes and myotomes
- <u>Pulses:</u> Brachial, radial and ulnar pulses

Root	Motor	Sensory	Reflex
C4	Scapular stabilization (winging)	Collar	
C5	Shoulder abduction Elbow flexion in supination	Lateral shoulder	Biceps
C6	Elbow flexion in neutral rotation, Wrist extension	Thumb	Brachioradialis
C7	Elbow extension Wrist flexion	Middle finger	Triceps
C8	Finger flexion, Hand grip Thumb extension	Little finger	
T1	Finger abduction	Upper chest & back	

Special tests

Muscle testing

a. Rotator cuff:

- <u>Supraspinatus</u>: Test both sides simultaneously –
    - ○ Elevate the shoulders in 90° elevation in scapular plane (30° forwards from coronal plane) in line with supraspinatus muscle + Apply downward pressure just above the elbow joint on arm (to reduce contribution of triceps in reinforcement of supraspinatus):
        - With thumb turned downwards/full internal rotation (Jobe's empty can test): Puts deltoid (another abductor) at mechanical disadvantage and supraspinatus at mechanical advantage (isolates supraspinatus)
        - With 45° external rotation (Full can test): Less painful and Same accuracy as empty can test

- Some authors prefer to test in only 30° elevation to reduce pain
    - Drop arm test: Passively abduct the shoulders to near full abduction and instruct the patient to drop their arms to the side in a controlled manner
        - Positive: Inability to maintain abduction or movement becomes jerky at 90-100° abduction (when supraspinatus starts to act)
- <u>Infraspinatus:</u>
    - Resisted external rotation in shoulder extension: Weakness in tear or dysfunction
    - Drop/lag sign: Release from passive maximal external rotation in extension (arm will fall in internal rotation if severe external rotator weakness)
- <u>Teres minor:</u>
    - Horn-blower test: Passively external rotate shoulder in 90° abduction in scapular plane, then release it asking the patient to maintain the position – forearm moves into neutral rotation (weakness of teres minor)

- <u>Subscapularis:</u>
    - Gerber's lift off test: In the position of "functional" internal rotation in extension – ask the patient to push the examiners hand from the small of the back (weakness - subscapularis weakness)
    - Lag sign: Similarly like in lift off test, passively move the hand of the patient away from the back and ask the patient to maintain this position (inability - weakness of subscapularis)
    - Napolean's or Belly-press test: Ask the patient to press the belly by bringing the elbow forwards from the plane of trunk; weakness of subscapularis results in –
        - Pectoralis major recruitment: Pulls the humerus & brings the elbow back
        - Compensatory movement: Wrist flexion
    - Bear hug test: Ask the patient to put the hand of the affected shoulder on top of the contralateral shoulder. Flex the shoulder to 90°. The examiner then tries to remove the hand from the shoulder (in an upward direction) while the patient is asked to continue to keep it there
        - Weakness/pain: Subscapularis dysfunction

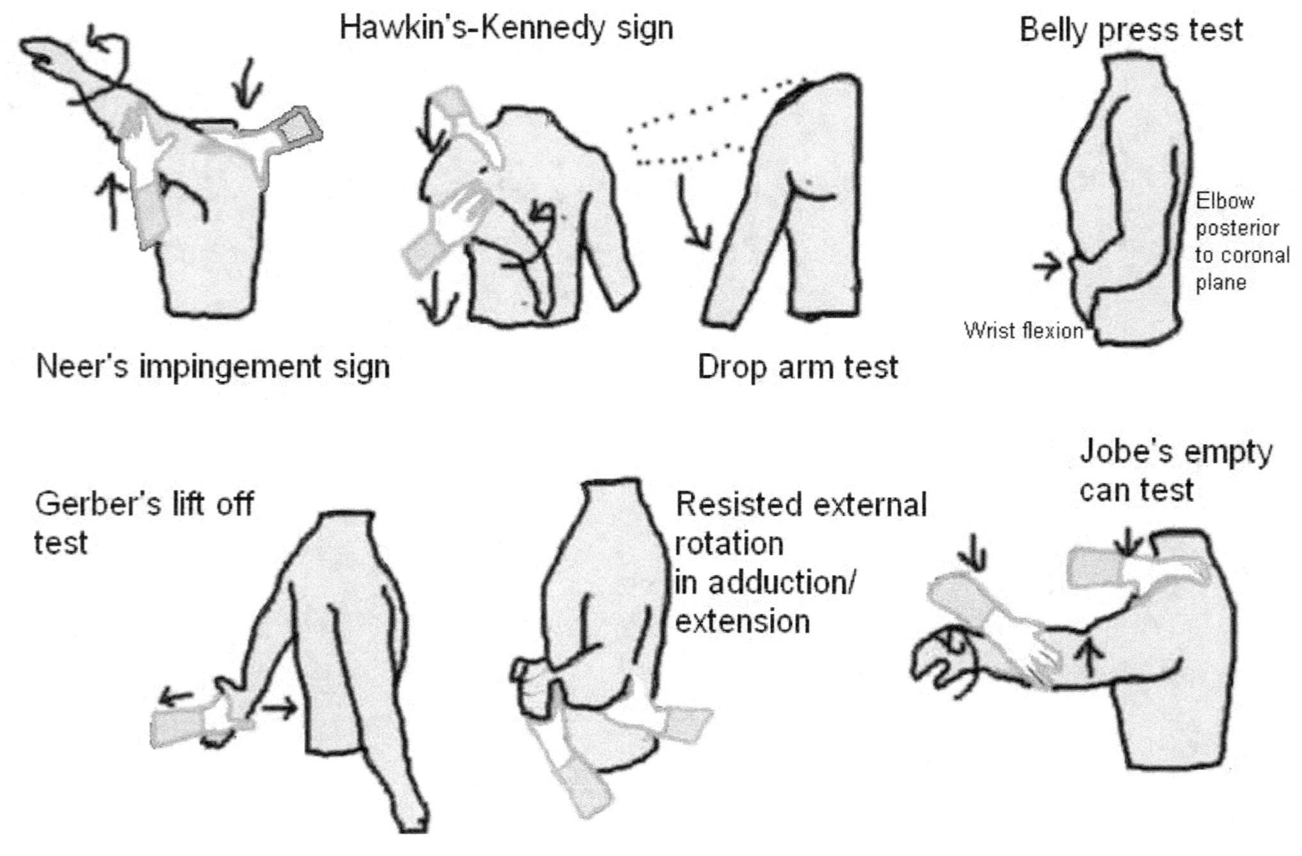

Hawkin's-Kennedy sign
Belly press test
Elbow
posterior
to coronal
plane
Wrist flexion
Neer's impingement sign
Drop arm test
Gerber's lift off
test
Resisted external
rotation
in adduction/
extension
Jobe's empty
can test

b. Other muscles around shoulder girdle:

- From front:
    - Deltoid: Abduction (middle fibers), Forward flexion (anterior fibers) or Extension (posterior fibers) against resistance
    - Pectoralis major: Palpate the muscles in anterior axillary folds when the patient squeezes in the waist with hands
    - Latissimus dorsi: Palpate the muscles in posterior axillary folds when the patient applies backward & downward pressure on your shoulders (like ladder climbing)
- From back:
    - Rhomboids: Feel the muscle between the scapulae when the patient pushes their elbows back against resistance (weakness leads to medial scapular winging = superomedial border of scapula moves medially)
    - Trapezius: Feel the muscle when the patient shrugs against resistance (weakness leads to lateral scapular winging

= superomedial border of scapular moves
laterally)

- Serratus anterior: Ask the patient to push
  the wall at shoulder-width, with the fingers
  & palm pointing downwards (weakness
  leads to medial scapular winging =
  superomedial border of scapula moves
  medially)

Impingement signs and Tests

a. Subacromial space:

- <u>Painful arc:</u> between 60-120° (as mentioned in
  MOVE)
- <u>Neer's impingement sign:</u> Passively abduct the
  internally rotated arm of patient in scapular plane
  with 1 hand while stabilizing the scapula with
  another hand
  - Positive: If pain is felt in the arc of 60-120°
- <u>Neer's impingement test:</u> If Neer's impingement
  sign is positive, repeat the test after instillation of
  local anesthetic in the subacromial space

- ○ Positive: If pain disappears
- <u>Hawkins-Kennedy test</u>: Passively abduct the arm to 90° in scapular plane with elbow flexed to 90° such that the forearm is parallel to the ground & from this position internal rotation is forced
  - ○ Positive: If pain is provoked

b. ACJ:

- <u>Scarf test/Cross-body adduction test</u>: Passively flex & adduct the internally rotated arm across the patient's body
  - ○ Positive: If pain is felt in ACJ and the pain disappears on repeat testing after 5-10 minutes of local anesthetic injection
- <u>Paxino's sign</u>: From the posterior, hook the thumb under the posterolateral margin of acromion & press in anterosuperior direction; at the same time push the clavicle inferiorly with index & middle finger (pain indicates osteoarthritis)

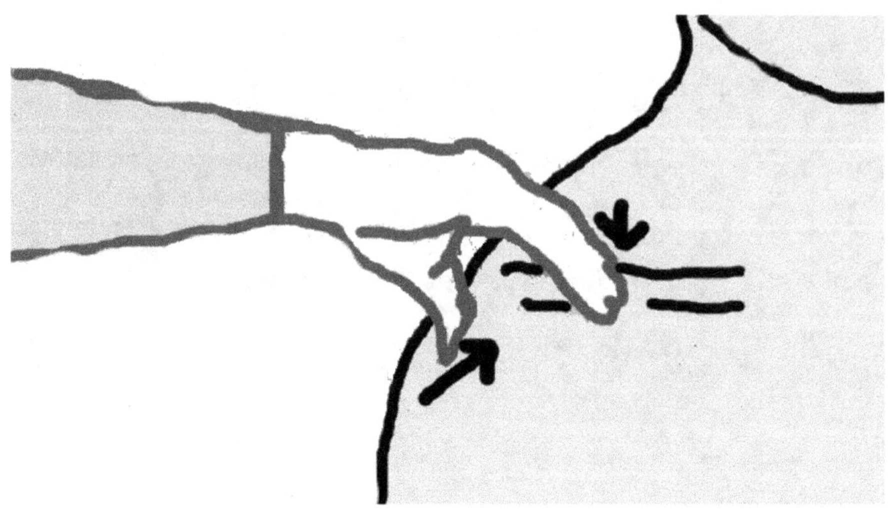

Paxino's sign

c. SLAP lesion (Injury to biceps tendon attachment in supraglenoid tubercle):

- <u>O'Brien's test:</u> The fully internally rotated arm (thumb pointing down) is forward flexed to 90° & adducted 15° (biceps tendon has tendency to slip out of bicipital groove & become unstable in medial direction due to lack of it's superior attachment) following which the patient is asked to resist the downward pressure applied over forearm by the examiner
    - Positive: Pain felt in Glenohumeral joint
        - Pain disappears with repeating the test with arm in full external

rotation (biceps tendon relocates back to the groove & is not dependent on it's superior attachment)

- <u>Crank test (like Apley's grinding test for knee menisci):</u> With arm in 160° of abduction in scapular plane apply an axial force with forced maximal internal and external rotation while stabilizing the scapula with other hand
    - Positive: Pain or click in Glenohumeral joint

d. Long head of biceps tendon (LHBT):

- <u>Speed's test:</u> Resisted forward flexion of shoulder with elbow fully extended & forearm supinated
    - Positive: Pain in bicipital groove area
- <u>Yergason's test:</u> Resisted supination of elbow held in 90° flexion with the arm by the side
    - Positive: Pain in bicipital groove area

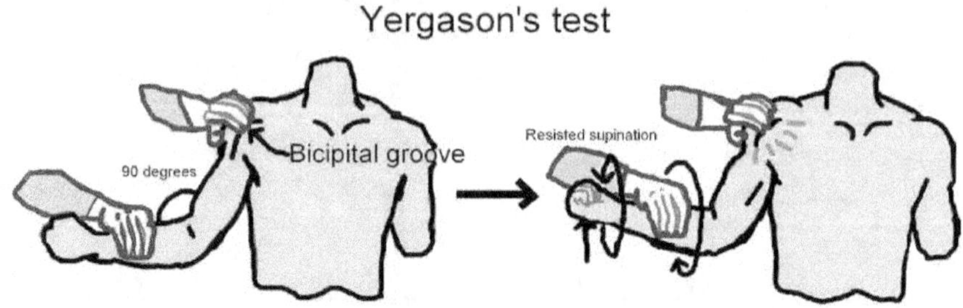

Laxity and Instability Assessment

a. Anterior & Posterior Shoulder Laxity:

- <u>Load & shift test:</u> Examiner stands behind the patient, stabilizes the scapula with one hand and with the other hand the examiner grasps the humeral head between their thumb & index finger to apply stress in anterior & posterior direction for anterior & posterior laxity respectively.

Hawkin's grade	Relation of humeral head to glenoid
Normal	Moves forward but doesn't sublux
I	Rides over glenoid rim (subluxes/doesn't dislocate)
II	Dislocates but spontaneously relocates
III	Dislocates & doesn't spontaneously relocate

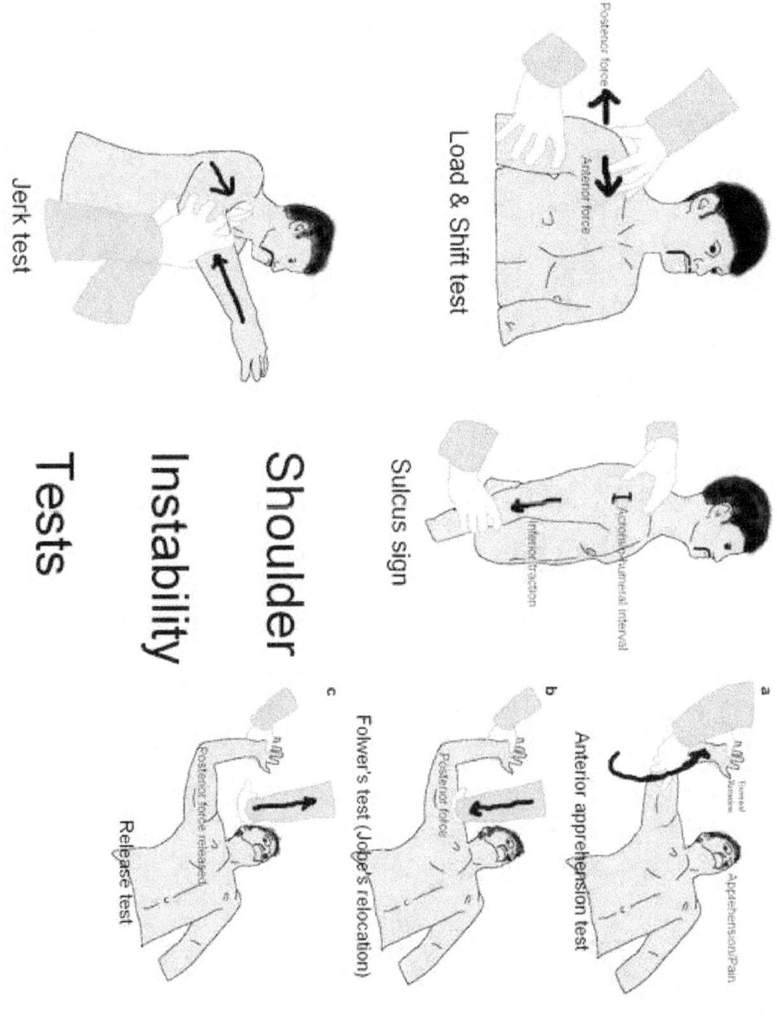

- <u>**Anterior & posterior drawer test:**</u> With the patient in supine position with shoulder in loose packed position (mild abduction, forward flexion &

external rotation i.e. wrist on the examiner's hip),
examiner stabilizes the scapula with one hand and
pulls & pushes the proximal humerus forward &
backward with another hand

- Grade according to Hawkin's classification
  like Load & shift test

b. Anterior glenohumeral instability:

- <u>Anterior apprehension test:</u> Stabilize the scapula
  (best performed lying or sitting on chair) with one
  hand and passively external rotate the arm
  abducted to 90° with elbow flexed 90° with or
  without anterior directed force (augmentation)
  - Positive: Patient experiences apprehension
    or discomfort
    - Anterior relocation test:
      Apprehension or discomfort is
      improved by posterior directed
      force on humeral head by the
      examiner
    - Release test: Subsequent sudden
      release of the anterior relocation

test aggravates the symptoms

again

- <u>Fulcrum test:</u> This is like the anterior apprehension test performed supine with the patient's scapula lying at the edge of the bed and the examiner places a fist under the glenohumeral joint while externally rotating the arm with another hand
    - Position: Patient experiences apprehension or discomfort

c. Posterior glenohumeral instability:

- <u>Posterior apprehension test (Jerk test):</u> Forward flex the patient's arm to 90° with elbow flexed to 90° in sitting position and apply posteriorly directed axial force on elbow while bringing the arm into adduction
    - Pain in glenohumeral joint = Posterior labral tear
    - Apprehension/pain = Subtle instability
    - Jerk/Jump = Instability

- - Relocation (felt): Passively abduct and externally rotate the arm maintaining the axial load
  - <u>Kim test:</u> It is the modification of Jerk test, in which the downward force displaces the humeral head more inferiorly (for posteroinferior labral tear and instability) –
    - Positive: Pain in posterior glenohumeral joint with or without clunk

d. Inferior shoulder laxity & instability:

- <u>Inferior sulcus sign:</u> Passive downward longitudinal traction on humerus in neutral rotation & observe for sulcus developing between acromion & humeral head laterally and grade according to acromio-humeral distance:
  - 1+: <1 cm
  - 2+: 1-2 cm (considered positive from here)
  - 3+: >2 cm translation
  - Test also positive when repeated in 30° external rotation: Additional incompetence of rotator interval structures

(coracohumeral ligament & superior glenohumeral ligament)

- ○ Instability: Pain, apprehension or symptoms of instability

- <u>Gagey hyperabduction test:</u> Passively abduct the patient's arm with elbow flexed 90° & forearm parallel to the ground until the scapula starts to move

  - ○ Laxity: Abduction >105° or more than 20° from opposite side

e. Generalized joint hyperlaxity: Beighton score

- Test if the patient has multi-directional instability
- <u>Positive:</u> ≥4 out of 9

Completion

1. Cervical spine and Thoracic outlet examination
2. Elbow examination

CHAPTER 11

Elbow Examination

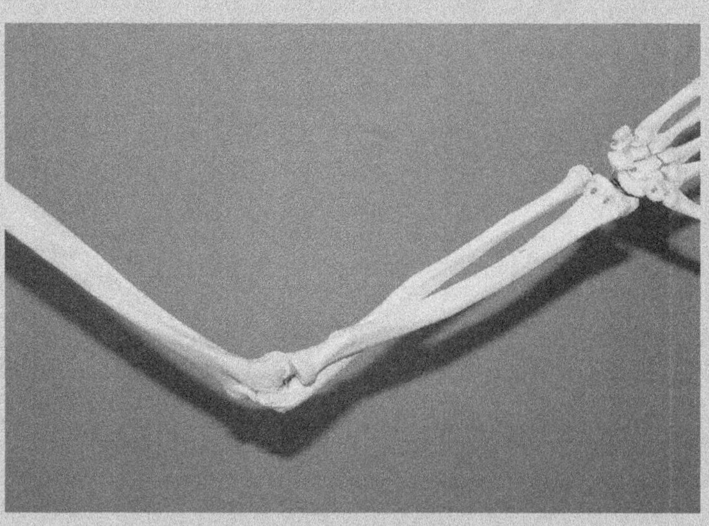

Elbow Examination

Elbow pathology can arise from any component of the joint including tendons, bursae, bones, or nerves. Tendinopathies (lateral and medial epicondylitis) can result from overuse in sports and activities of daily living. Rheumatoid (inflammatory), post-traumatic, and primary osteoarthritis are three primary patterns of arthritis affecting the elbow.

Exposure

Exposed from the shoulders down to the hands (bilateral)

Inspection (Look)

Look for **SEADS** & carefully compare both sides.

From anterior

1. Elbows fully extended and forearm supinated (if not

   possible, assessment of carrying angle cannot be done):

Observe carrying angle (between long axis of arm and forearm)

   a. <u>Normal:</u> Average 10° in males and 15° in females

   b. <u>Neutral:</u> Cubitus rectus

   c. <u>Increased carrying angle:</u> Cubitus valgus

   d. <u>Decreased carrying angle:</u> Cubitus varus (gunstock deformity)

2. Elbows in full flexion: Look for biceps tendon prominence, deformities and bony prominences

   a. Elbow changes from valgus to varus during flexion in normal conditions (brings hand to face)

   b. Common swellings:

       i.   <u>Tip of olecranon:</u> Olecranon bursitis

       ii. <u>Olecranon and subcutaneous border of ulna:</u> Rheumatoid nodule

From lateral

1. Look for limitation of terminal extension or hyperextension

2. Lateral epicondylar prominence

3. Any abnormality in brachioradialis and long extensors of elbow

From posterior

1. Triceps bulge
2. Olecranon
3. Paraolecranon depression (fullness indicates joint effusion)
4. Infracondylar recess just distal to lateral epicondyle (fullness indicates joint effusion)
5. Ulna

Palpation (Feel)

Superficial

- Temperature
- Superficial tenderness

Deep

Lateral

1. Lateral supracondylar ridge
2. Lateral epicondyle
   a. <u>Pain over ECRB attachment</u> (few mm distal & anterior to tip of lateral epicondyle) = Lateral epicondylitis or Tennis elbow
   b. Perform <u>provocative tests</u> (if lateral epicondylitis suspected):
      i. Pain reproduced at lateral epicondyle by resisted wrist extension with elbow fully extended & pronated
      ii. Cozen's test: Pain reproduced at lateral epicondyle by resisted wrist extension & radial deviation with the elbow flexed & forearm pronated
      iii. Maudsley test: Pain reproduced at lateral epicondyle by resisted extension of middle finger

iv. Mill's test: Pain reproduced at lateral epicondyle by passive volar flexion of wrist with forearm pronated & elbow extended

v. Chair test: Pain reproduced at lateral epicondyle by lifting the chair with elbow extended forearm pronated & shoulder forward flexed

3. Common extensor origin

4. Lateral collateral ligament

5. Capitellar joint line

   a. Tenderness = Articular injury or Osteochondritis dissecans

6. Infracondylar recess (between lateral condyle & radial head)

   a. <u>Boggy swelling</u> = Synovial hypertrophy

   b. <u>Fluctuation</u> = Intra-articular fluid

7. Radial head (appreciated during pronation & supination; should align with capitellum in all positions of elbow & forearm)

   a. <u>Radial head doesn't align with capitellum</u> = Congenital or post-traumatic dislocation

b. <u>Tenderness, pain on rotation movement &</u>
   <u>crepitus</u> = Radial head fracture or
   Radio-capitellar degenerative disease

8. Forearm

   a. Tenderness over radial nerve about <u>3-5 cm</u>
      <u>distal to lateral epicondyle</u> = Radial tunnel
      syndrome (RTS)

   b. Perform <u>provocative tests</u> (if RTS
      suspected):

      i. Pain reproduced at radial tunnel
         with resisted middle finger
         extension (similar to Maudsley's
         test)

      ii. Pain reproduced at radial tunnel
          with resisted supination with elbow
          & wrist in extension

      iii. Pain reproduced at radial tunnel
           with passive pronation & wrist
           flexion

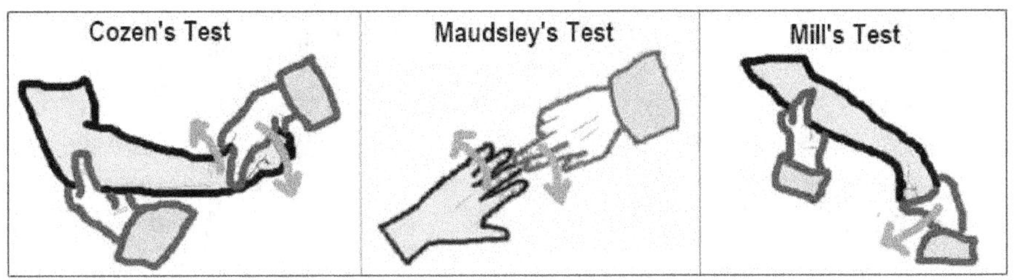

Provocative tests for lateral epicondylitis

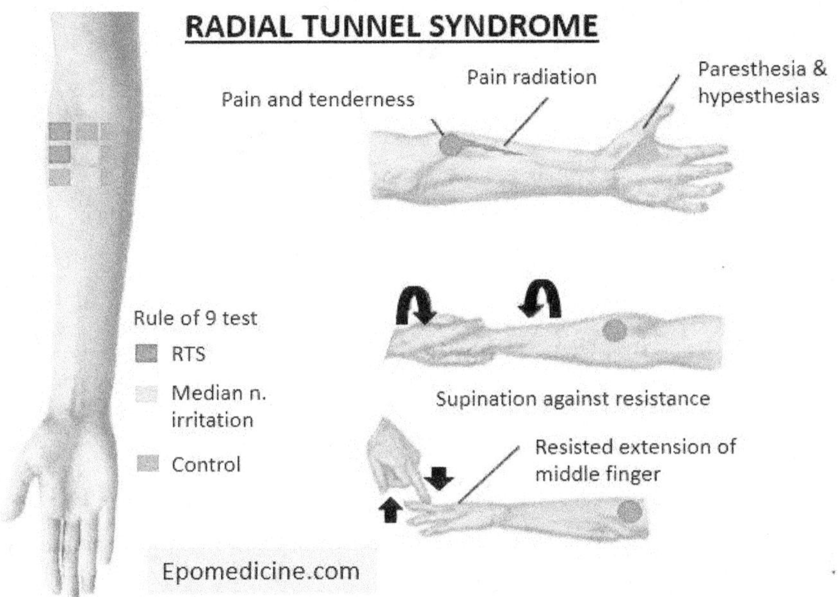

Provocative tests for radial tunnel syndrome

Anterior

From lateral to medial:

1. Brachioradialis

2. Biceps tendon

a. <u>Hook test:</u> Hook the finger around lateral edge of biceps tendon while the patient actively flexes the elbow & supinates the forearm

   i. Normal or partially torn tendon = Tendon can be hooked 1 cm beneath

   ii. Rupture of biceps tendon insertion = Inability to hook the tendon

3. Brachial artery

4. Median nerve

5. Pronator teres

   a. Tenderness at <u>belly of pronator teres</u> = Pronator syndrome

   b. Perform provocative tests (if pronator syndrome suspected):

      i. <u>Tinel sign</u> in proximal anterior forearm (symptoms reproduced in median nerve distribution

      ii. <u>Resisted elbow flexion with forearm supination</u> (compression at bicipital aponeurosis)

iii. <u>Resisted forearm pronation with elbow extended</u> (compression at two heads of pronator teres)

iv. <u>Resisted contraction of FDS to middle finger</u> (compression at FDS fibrous arch)

Myositis ossificans may be palpable as bony hard swelling.

Medial

1. Medial supracondylar line:

    a. <u>Epitrochlear lymph nodes</u> (drains ulnar forearm & hand): Lateral and about 3 cm superior to medial epicondyle in a groove between biceps and triceps muscle

2. Medial epicondyle & common flexor origin

    a. <u>Tenderness 5-10 mm distal & anterior to tip of medial epicondyle</u> = Medial epicondylitis or Golfer's elbow

    b. Perform <u>provocative tests</u> (if medial epicondylitis suspected):

i. Reverse Cozen's test: Pain reproduced at medial epicondyle with resisted wrist flexion

ii. Pain reproduced at medial epicondyle with passive extension of wrist & elbow

iii. No instability or apprehension with valgus stress or milking maneuver (to differentiate from MCL injury)

3. Ulnar nerve (between medial epicondyle & olecranon)

a. May sublux anteriorly during flexion in 10%

b. Roll between the fingers:

i. <u>Normal:</u> round, soft and tubular

ii. <u>Leprosy:</u> thickened

c. Check for <u>Tinel's sign</u> (by gentle percussion of nerve)

d. Perform <u>provocative tests</u> (if cubital tunnel syndrome suspected):

i. Elbow flexion test: Paresthesia in ulnar nerve distribution by active full flexion of elbow with forearm in supination & wrist extension for >60 seconds (upto 3 minutes)

    ii. Jeanne sign: Compensatory thumb MCP hyperextension & thumb adduction by EPL (radial nerve) with key pinch

    iii. Wartenberg's sign: Persistent little finger abduction and extension during attempted adduction secondary to weak intrinsics and unopposed action of EDM

    iv. Masse sign: Palmar arch flattening and loss of ulnar hand elevation secondary to weak opponens digiti quinti and decreased small finger MCP flexion

4. Medial collateral ligament (just inferior to medial epicondyle with elbow at 50-70° flexion to move flexor-pronator mass anteriorly)

    a. <u>Tenderness</u> = MCL injury

Elbow flexion test

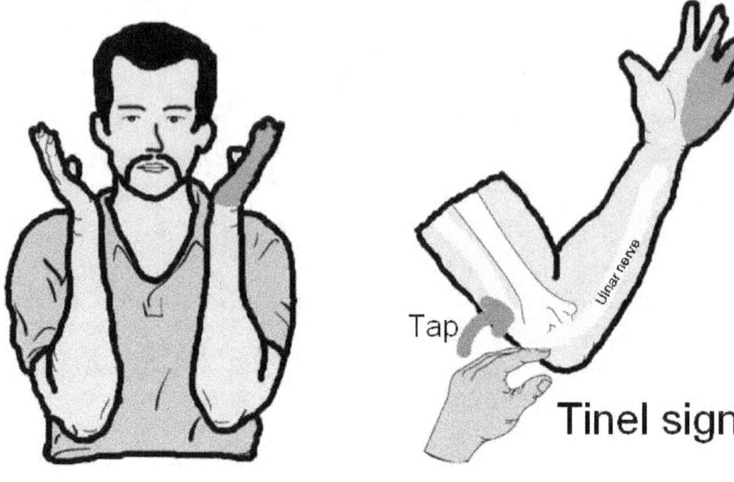

Provocation tests for ulnar nerve

Posterior

1. Olecranon:

    a. <u>In extension:</u> Lateral epicondyle, olecranon & medial epicondyle must form a straight line

    b. <u>In flexion:</u> Lateral epicondyle, olecranon & medial epicondyle must form an isosceles triangle

    c. <u>Abnormal arrangement</u> of these structures = Elbow dislocation

    d. <u>Tenderness at posteromedial olecranon</u> = Valgus extension overload (Pitcher's elbow)

i. <u>Provocative test:</u> Valgus extension overload test

1. The elbow is rapidly extended while a valgus stress is applied, causing impingement of the posteromedial tip of the olecranon on the medial wall of the olecranon fossa.

2. In elbow extension: Triceps insertion

a. <u>Focal tenderness</u> = Triceps insertionitis (tendonitis)

b. Perform <u>provocative maneuver </u>(if triceps insertionitis suspected):

i. Reproduction of pain at triceps insertion with resisted elbow extension

c. <u>Swelling, ecchymosis +/- palpable defect</u> = May be due to triceps tendon rupture

d. Perform <u>provocative maneuver</u> (if triceps tendon rupture suspected):

i. Inability to extend elbow against resistance (some patients can

extend the elbow if lateral
expansion & anconeus is intact)

ii.   Modified Thompson squeeze test:
Inability to extend elbow against
the gravity with the patient lying
down prone with elbow on the
edge of table and forearm hanging
down (indicates ruptured lateral
expansion and triceps tendon)

3. In 30° elbow flexion: Olecranon fossa

a. Loose body may be palpable here

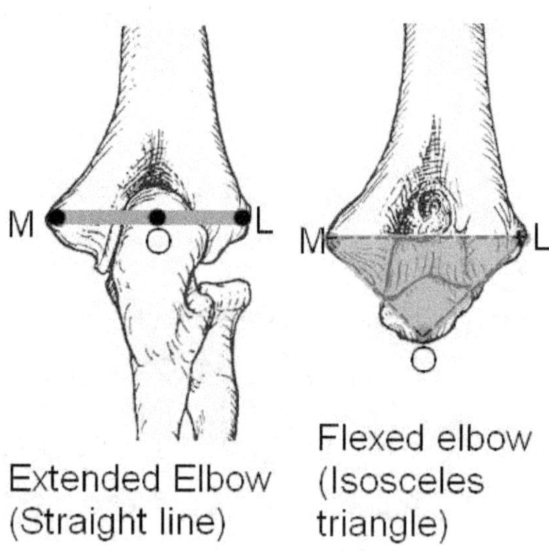

Extended Elbow
(Straight line)

Flexed elbow
(Isosceles
triangle)

Olecranon bursa or rheumatoid nodules may be present.

Move

Instruct the patient to perform active movements and then perform passive movements over it to see if there are any discrepancies between the two.

Note the smoothness of movement and the endpoint:

- <u>Soft endpoint:</u> Effusion or capsular tightness
- <u>Firm endpoint:</u> Mechanical block (loose body, fracture, osteophyte)

Move	Technique	Range	Comments	End feel
Flexion	Both forearms supinated, Both shoulders abducted to 90°	0-140°	Functional = 100°	Soft
Extension	Both forearms supinated, Both shoulders abducted to 90°	Up to -10°	Loss of full extension = intra articular pathology	Hard

| Supination | Both elbows flexed to 90° & arms adducted (prevents compensatory shoulder movement) with the fist holding pen/pencil or "thumbs up" | 0-85° | Functional = 45° | Firm |
| Pronation | Both elbows flexed to 90° & arms adducted (prevents compensatory shoulder movement) with the fist holding pen/pencil or "thumbs up" | 0-75° | Functional = 45° | Firm |

Measure

1. **Lengths:**

- <u>Arm:</u> Posterolateral corner of acromion to lateral epicondyle
- <u>Forearm:</u> Lateral epicondyle to radial styloid
- <u>Triangle formed by lateral epicondyle, olecranon & medial epicondyle:</u>
    - Inter-epicondylar distance
    - Olecranon tip to medial epicondyle
    - Olecranon tip to lateral epicondyle

2. **Carrying angle:** Measured with goniometer between:

- <u>Arm axis:</u> Midpoint between anterior axillary fold-lateral deltoid bulge to midpoint of inter-epicondylar line of humerus
- <u>Forearm axis:</u> Midpoint of inter-epicondylar line of humerus to midpoint of inter-styloid line of wrist

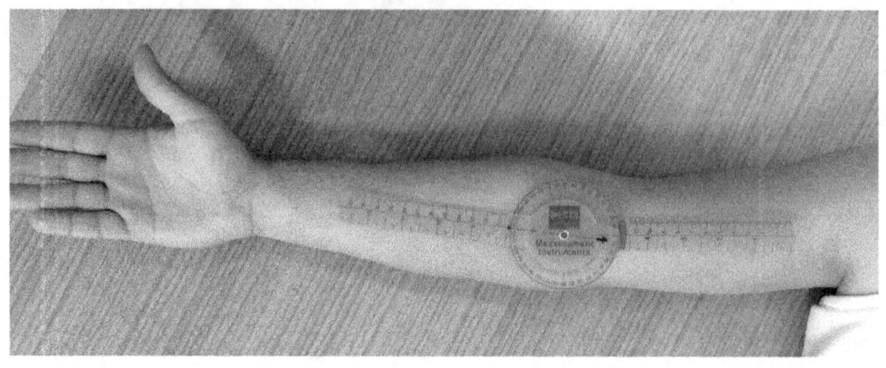

Evaluation of the Elbow Carrying Angle in Healthy Individuals - Scientific Figure on ResearchGate. Available from: https://www.researchgate.net/figure/Showing-the-measurement-o f-the-carrying-angle_fig1_324231462 [CC BY 4.0]

3. **Circumference:**

- <u>Mid-arm circumference:</u> Measured at midpoint of the arm length
- <u>Forearm circumference:</u> Usually measured 7 cm below the medial epicondyle (at the level of maximum muscular girth)

4. **Rotational deformities:** Rotation deformities occur due to abnormality of shoulder or elbow –

- <u>Asymmetric rotation of shoulder:</u> Measure internal and external rotation of shoulder in 90°

abduction & arms by the side (adduction) and compare with another side

- o Internal rotation deformity at elbow results in –
    - Restricted shoulder external rotation
    - Complementary increased shoulder internal rotation
- o Fallacies:
    - For this test to be useful the deformity must be unilateral, and shoulder must be normal
    - Dominant shoulder has increased physiological rotation

- <u>Yamamoto technique:</u>
  - o With the elbow flexed to 90°, shoulder in full extension & forearm behind the back, the patient bends forwards
  - o Examiner lifts the forearm maximally away from the back, resulting in maximal internal rotation
    - Forearm parallel to the ground: No internal rotation deformity

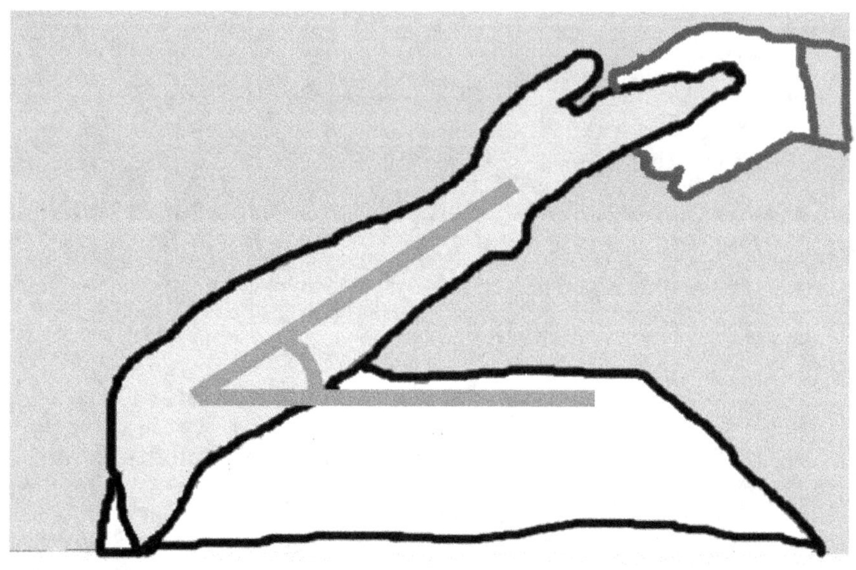

Angle the forearm makes against the ground (horizontal line) is the internal rotation deformity (Yamamoto method)

Neurovascular Examination

1. Neurologic:

- C5-T1 myotome, dermatome and reflexes
- Peripheral nerves (median, ulnar and radial nerves)

Nerve	Entrapment sites	Comments
a. Median nerve (C5-T1)	Struther's ligament (Supracondylar process syndrome)	Weakness in pronator teres & all distal muscles supplied Sensory loss in median nerve distribution
	Between heads of pronator teres (Pronator syndrome)	Similar to Supracondylar process syndrome but pronator teres is spared
	Between heads of pronator teres (AIN syndrome)	Sensation spared OK sign
b. Ulnar nerve (C8, T1)	Cubital tunnel	Weakness and sensory loss in ulnar nerve distribution
c. Radial nerve (C5-T1)	Fibrous band in supinator or arcade of Frohse (PIN syndrome)	Wrist & finger drop Sensations spared
	Inside supinator, i.e. radial tunnel syndrome)	Mimics lateral epicondylitis
	Under brachioradialis tendon (Cheiralgia paresthetica or Wartenberg's disease)	Nocturnal pain along dorsum of wrist, thumb & 1st webspace

2. **Vascular:** Brachial artery, Radial artery, Ulnar artery

Special tests

Valgus Stability

1. **Valgus stress test:**

- Elbow flexed to 30° (to unlock olecranon from the olecranon fossa and relax the anterior capsule)
- Arm fully externally rotated (to stabilize the shoulder)
- Apply valgus force with 1 hand while palpating MCL with another hand
- <u>Opening of joint + Local pain/tenderness (compared to other side):</u> MCL Injury

2. **O'Brien's test (milking maneuver):** Hold the patient's thumb with 1 hand and fully flex the elbow while applying a valgus stress with another hand on MCL (tests posterior band of MCL)

- <u>Apprehension + Opening of joint</u> = MCL injury
- <u>Pain at site of MCL</u> = Partial MCL tear without gross instability

Varus instability

Varus stress test:

- Elbow flexed to 30° (to unlock olecranon from the olecranon fossa and relax the anterior capsule)
- Arm fully internally rotated (to stabilize the shoulder)
- Apply varus force with 1 hand while palpating lateral joint line
- <u>Opening of joint + Local pain/tenderness (compared to other side):</u> LCL injury

PLRI

Posterolateral rotatory instability (PLRI) test tests integrity of LUCL (Lateral Ulnar Collateral Ligament).

Apprehension signs:

1. <u>Chair push-up test:</u> When patient is instructed to stand from chair using their arms to push them up, the patient is reluctant to extend elbow fully (produces maneuver similar to lateral pivot shift test – axial load, valgus and supination)

2. <u>Floor push-up test:</u> Patient is reluctant to extend elbow fully due to similar forces applied

3. <u>Table top relocation test:</u>
    a. 1st part: patient places hand of symptomatic elbow around edge of table and is asked to perform press-up maneuver with elbow pointing laterally and forearm supinated
        i. pain and apprehension at 40° flexion: positive test
    b. 2nd part: same maneuver as 1st part but examiner places thumb over patient's radial head during the maneuver to prevent radial head subluxation

i. relief of pain and apprehension: positive test

ii. pain: intra-articular radial head fracture

Lateral pivot shift test (O'Driscoll):

- Patient lies supine with shoulder fully flexed & externally rotated, elbow flexed
- Examiner holds the patient's forearm & wrist
- Axial compression and valgus force is applied to patient's elbow while slowly supinating the forearm and extending the elbow
- <u>Positive test indicates PLRI (Posterolateral rotatory instability):</u>
  - At 40° flexion (supination is reduced & only a pure valgus torque is maintained): Radio-capitellar *subluxation/dislocation* occurs leading to a prominence postero-laterally and a dimple between the radial head and the capitellum.
  - Further flexion >40° flexion: This subluxation/dislocation suddenly *reduces* which may be accompanied by

palpable/visible clunk (*triceps tension reduces the radial head*)

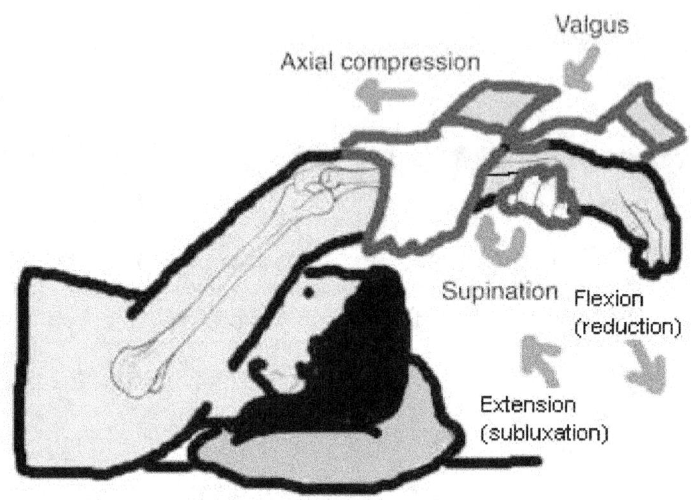

Pivot shift test for elbow

VPMRI

Varus Posteromedial Rotatory Instability (VPMRI) is usually associated with anteromedial (AM) facet coronoid fracture & disruption of lateral ligamentous complex.

1. **Gravity varus stress test (can be done in clinic):**

- Patient is instructed to keep shoulder in 90° abduction and forearm in neutral rotation (palm faces ground)
- Patient actively moves elbow in flexion & extension

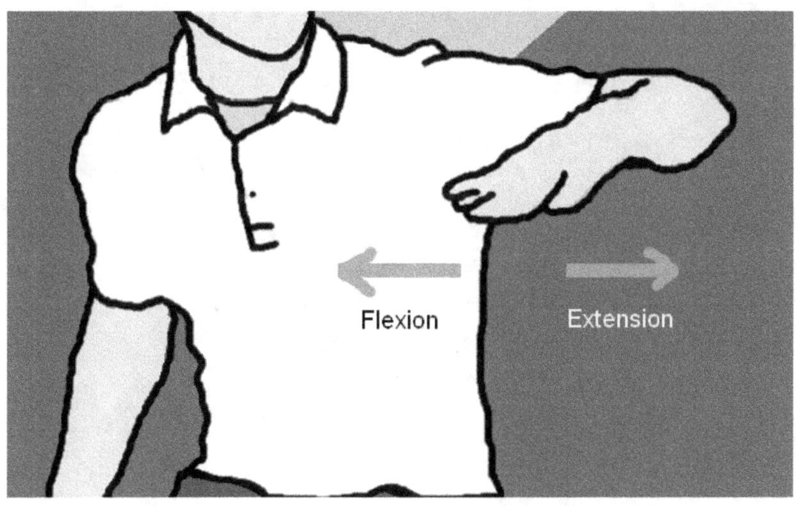

Pain/Crepitus/Instability = Positive test

2. **Hyperpronation test (under anesthesia):** Passive pronation at 90° elbow flexion produces palpable ulnohumeral subluxation.

Impingement tests

1. **Posterior elbow impingement:** Gentle rapid passive hyperextension induces posterior elbow pain

- Olecranon tip osteophyte on olecranon fossa
- Olecranon fossa loose bodies on olecranon tip

2. **Anterior elbow impingement:** Gentle rapid passive hyperflexion induces anterior elbow pain

- Coronoid process osteophyte on coronoid fossa
- Radial head on radial fossa osteophyte

Completion

1. **Shoulder & forearm** examination (for compensations & consequences of elbow pathology)
2. **Wrist & hand** examination (common flexor & extensor tendons around elbow crosses wrist & small joints of hand)

CHAPTER 12

Wrist Examination

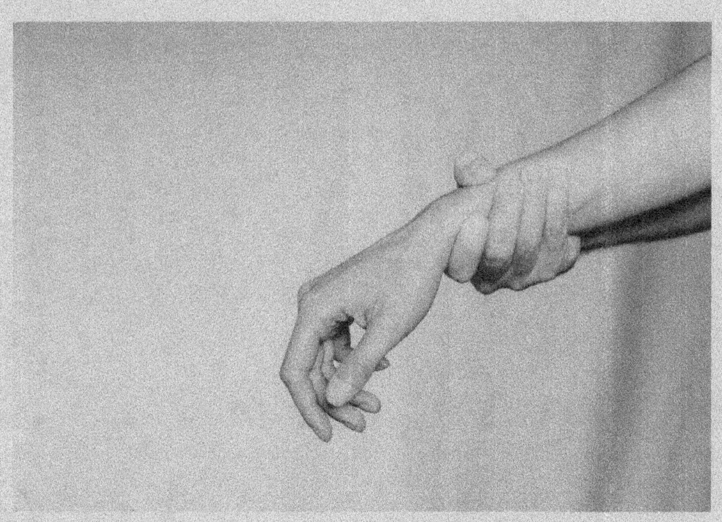

Wrist Examination

Clinical examination of the wrist can be problematic, due to the large number of structures that are found in a confined space, which give rise to a wide range of pathologies. Hence, it is essential for clinicians to develop a thorough and systematic technique of examination to list out possible differential diagnoses and reach a proper provisional diagnosis.

Exposure

Expose to above the elbows. Examine both hands side by side.

Look

Both dorsal and palmar aspects of the wrist. Follow **SEADS**.

Some important points:

- **Rheumatoid hand**

- Shoulder sign: Outline of thumb will form a step if subluxation of CMC joint >2-3 mm

- Radial malunion: radial shortening and prominence of ulna

- Madelung's deformity: volar bowing of distal radius with dorsal prominence of ulna

- Dorsal wrist ganglion: overlie scapholunate ligament; just distal to Lister's tubercle

- Carpal boss (bony swelling at 2nd & 3rd CMC level): more distal than simple ganglion

- Extensor digitorum brevis manus (accessory muscle): distal to extensor retinaculum (moves with finger extension)

- Volar ganglion

Feel

Follow **TEST Areas**.

Areas of emphasis: Follow a sequence (Start dorsal-radial and move in a circle around wrist) –

a. <u>Dorsal:</u>

1. Thumb CMC (1st metacarpal base and trapezium)
2. Anatomical snuff box (between EPB/APL, i.e. 1st extensor compartment and EPL): Scaphoid in floor
3. Radial styloid
   a. Just proximal to radial styloid: DeQuervain's tenosynovitis
   b. 1-2 cm proximal to radial styloid: Superficial branch of radial nerve
4. Distal radius
5. Lister's tubercle
   a. Radial side: ECRL and ECRB (2nd extensor compartment)
   b. Ulnar side: EPL (3rd extensor compartment)
   c. 5 cm proximal to radial styloid: Intersection syndrome (intersection of 1st and 2nd extensor compartment)
6. Scapholunate interval:

a. Lunate: just distal to dorsal rim of radius in line with 3rd metacarpal

b. Scapholunate interval: valley between dorsal pole of lunate and proximal pole of scaphoid

7. DRUJ

8. 4th (EDC and EIP) and 5th (EDM) extensor compartments

9. TFCC

10. Ulnar styloid

11. Ulnar snuffbox (between ECU and FCU)

12. Fovea (TFCC): between ulnar styloid and pisiform

13. Clinical ulnar variance: measured between ulnar styloid (opposed to articular surface in true ulnar variance) and radial styloid (radial styloid is slightly distal than ulnar styloid normally)

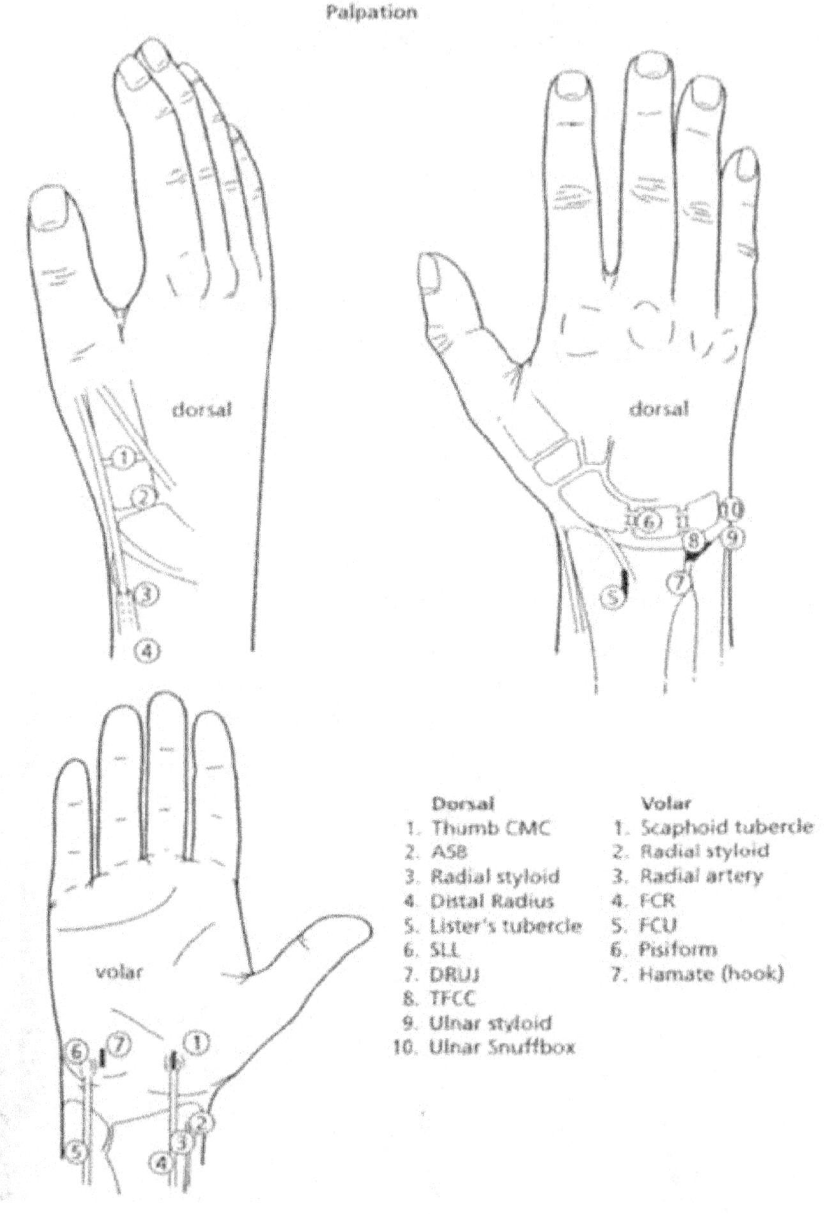

Source: Hand and Wrist Examination – WikiMSK [CC BY-SA 4.0]

b. <u>Volar:</u>

1. Scaphoid tubercle
2. Radial styloid
3. Radial artery
4. FCR, Palmaris longus and carpal tunnel & FCU
5. Pisiform: within tendon of FCU
6. Hamate (hook): slightly distal and radial to the pisiform bone

Move

Test passive then active movements.

1. Dorsiflexion: 0-70 degrees
2. Palmar flexion: 0-80 degrees
3. Radial deviation: 0-20 degrees
4. Ulnar deviation: 0-30 degrees
5. Pronation: 75 degrees
6. Supination: 80 degrees

Measure

Measure grip strength using:

1. Dynamometer or

2. Sphygmomanometer: First, the sphygmomanometer is rolled into a cylinder comfortable for the patient to grip at rest. The cuff is then inflated to 20 mmHg, and the patient applies maximal grip force to the cuff. The gauge needle indicates the patient's applied pressure (must increase by at least 150 mmHg).

Neurovascular examination

Test the muscles and nerves. Do not forget to perform Allen's test.

Modified Allen's test:

1. Ask patient to clench fist and the examiner occludes ulnar and radial artery.

2. Patient is asked to release fist after 30 seconds.

3. Hand should remain blanched (if not, the pressure applied by examiner is inadequate).

4. Release occlusion of ulnar artery to check ulnar artery and radial artery to check radial artery.

5. Hand must flush within 5-15 seconds.

Special tests

Condition	Site	Test	Technique & Interpretation
De Quervain's disease	Radial	Finkelstein	1st: Ask to ulnar deviate wrist actively 2nd: Then passively tuck thumb in fist
		Eichoff's	Ask to actively tuck thumb in fist and passively ulnar deviate wrist
Intersection syndrome	Radial	Resisted wrist extension and thumb extension	Increased pain over intersection site

Scapholu nate instability	Radial	Scaphoid shift test (Kirk-Wats on)	Examiner places index finger over SL interval and thumb presses over scaphoid tubercle. With another hand, the wrist is deviated from ulnar into radial deviation. The thumb pressure over scaphoid tubercle resists palmar deviation of scaphoid during radial deviation, which would lead to dorsal subluxation of scaphoid over distal radius dorsal lip in SL instability ("click"). It is positive in upto 36% of normal individuals (esp. with laxity)
Midcarpal instability	Centr al	Midcarpal shift test (Lichtman)	Examiner stabilizes forearm with one hand. With other hand, examiner puts thumb over capitate dorsally. A volar directed force is applied as the wrist is ulnar deviated. A palpable clunk is felt (catch-up movement of proximal carpal row which is slow to dorsiflex in midcarpal instability as the wrist is ulnar deviated)

Ulnar sided pathology – general	Ulnar	Ulnocarpal stress test	Axial load to the wrist held in ulnar deviation and neutral flexion/extension. The forearm is then rotated. A positive test elicits pain on the ulnar side of the wrist.
Lunotriqu etral instability	Ulnar	Ballotteme nt test (Reagan)	Thumb and index finger of one hand fixes lunate. Triquetrum is displaced with thumb and index finger of another hand into dorsal and volar direction. Positive test is indicated by laxity, pain or crepitus.
		Kleinman Shear test (Shuck test)	Stabilize by pinching lunate with one hand. Apply shear to lunotriquetral joint by applying force on pisiform volarly to push it dorsally (indirect shear on lunotriquetral through piso-triquetral joint). Pain or clicking indicates positive test.
Pisotrique tral arthritis	Ulnar	Pisotriquet ral Grind test	Pisiform is held between the thumb and index finger. Compression is applied and the pisiform displaced back and

			forth in a radial and ulnar direction.
DRUJ	Ulnar	DRUJ Compression test	The examiner compresses the radial and ulnar heads together and then rotates the forearm.
		Piano key test	Stabilize the forearm and press the ulna with thumb. Increased excursion suggests dorsal subluxation of ulna.
		Radioulnar drawer test	Radius is stabilised with one hand. The ulna is grasped between the fingers and thumb of the other hand and moved dorsally and volarly.
		Dimple sign	Longitudinal traction is applied across the wrist. A force is applied to the dorsal aspect of the ulna shaft. If a 'dimple' appears at the level of the DRUJ, then this suggests volar subluxation.
TFCC	Ulnar	TFCC Compression test	With elbow flexed and rested on table, stabilize forearm with one hand and grasp the fingers with other hand. Wrist is loaded and

			moved in radial and ulnar deviation.
		TFCC grind test	Wrist dorsiflexion, axial load, ulnar deviation, and rotation. Pain and crepitus are elicited.
ECU subluxation	Ulnar	Supination, ulnar deviation and dorsiflexion	Painful subluxation of ECU

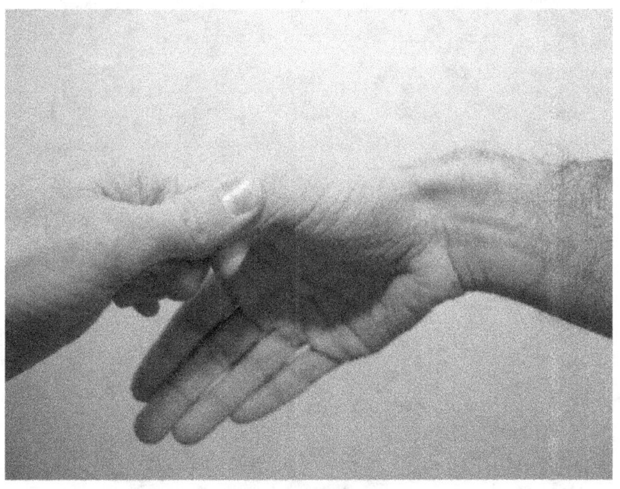

Finkelstein test

PhilippN, CC BY-SA 3.0, via Wikimedia Commons

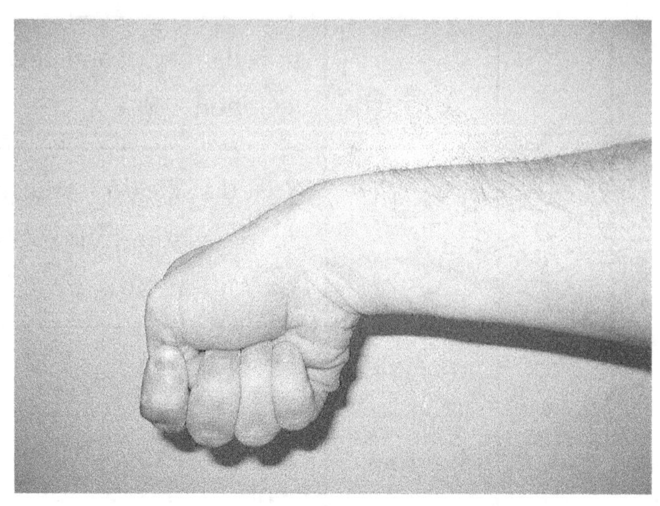

Eichoff's test

InvictaHOG at English Wikipedia, Public domain, via Wikimedia Commons

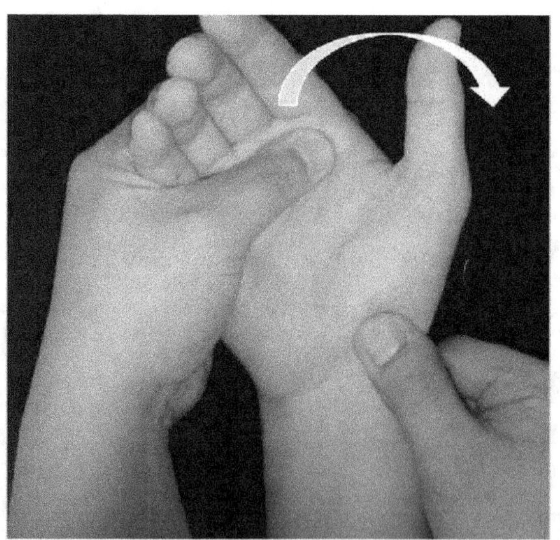

Watson (scaphoid shift) test

Chae, Seungbum & Roh, Youn-Tae & Park, Il-Jung. (2020). Scapholunate Dissociation: Current Concepts of the Treatments. Archives of Hand and Microsurgery. 25. 10.12790/ahm.20.0013. [CC-BY-4]

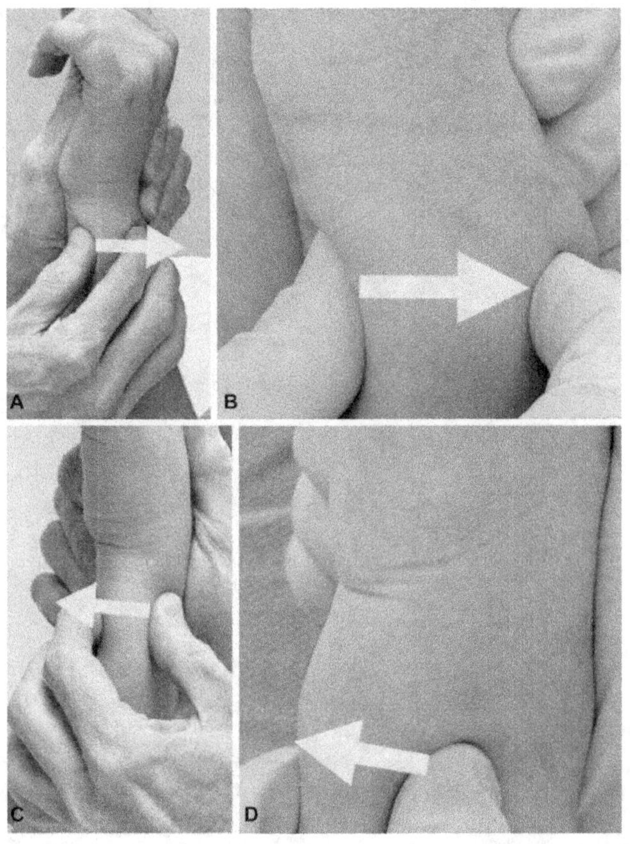

Stress test for DRUJ

Bachinskas, Andrew & Helsper, Elizabeth & Morris, Harry & Hearon, Bernard. (2019). Nonsurgical Treatment for Acute Posttraumatic Distal Radioulnar Joint Instability: A Case Series. Journal of Hand Surgery Global Online. 2. 10.1016/j.jhsg.2019.10.002.

CHAPTER 13

Hand Examination

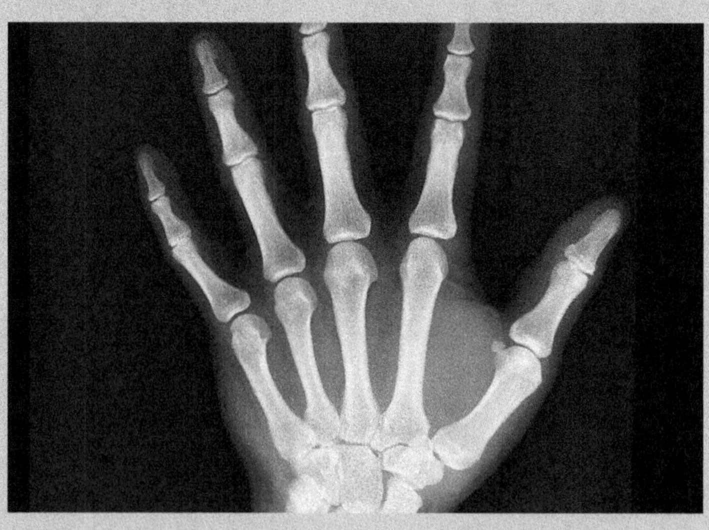

Hand Examination

The hands have a higher concentration of joints than any other part of the body. A general examination of the hand includes inspection, palpation, assessment of range of motion, and assessment of grip strength.

Look

Examine **SEADS** with palms facing upwards and downwards:

- Nails:
  - Subungual exostosis
  - Glomus tumor (bluish tinge)
  - Ganglion cyst at nail bed (grooved nail)
  - Psoriatic arthropathy (pitting and onycholysis)
- Swellings:
  - <u>Volar:</u>
    - Inclusion dermoid cysts

- - - Ganglion of A1 pulley (Pearl ganglion)
    - GCT of flexor sheath (usually in relation to proximal phalanx)
  - Dorsal:
    - DIP: Heberden's node, Mucous cyst
    - PIP: Bouchard's node, Garrod's pad
    - MCP: Rheumatoid nodule
    - CMC (index and middle finger): Carpal boss
- Attitude:
  - Palm upwards: Gradual cascade of fingers (increasing flexion in joints from index to little finger)
  - Palm downwards: Gradual cascade of fingers (increasing extension in joints from little to index finger)
  - Tenodesis effect of wrist movement
- Puckering and ridging/pitting and nodules of skin in the palm sometimes extending into finger: Dupuytren's contracture
- Deformity: Look for rheumatoid hand deformities, clawing, angular and rotational deformities

Interrupted finger cascade = Tendon divided or stuck

Normal finger cascade but absent active motion = Nerve injury

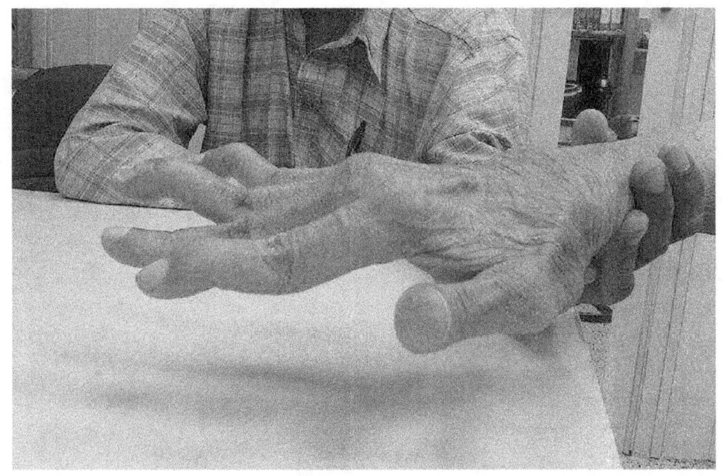

Rheumatoid hand – Swan neck deformity

User:Phoenix119, CC BY-SA 3.0, via Wikimedia Commons

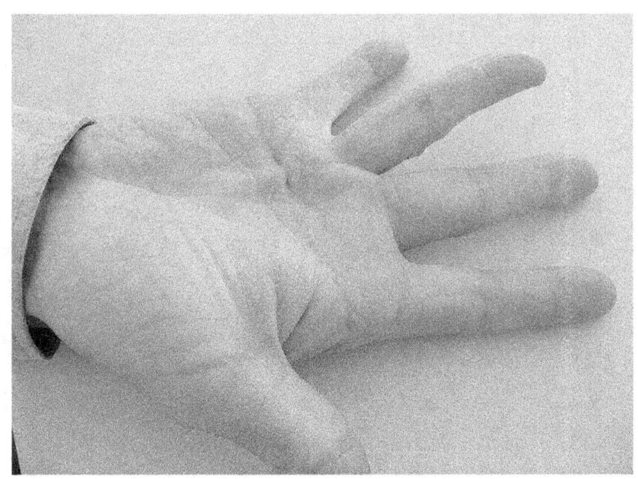

Dupuytren's contracture of ring finger

Frank C. Müller, CC BY-SA 4.0, via Wikimedia Commons

Feel

Examine **TEST Areas**

- Anhidrosis: Nerve damage

- Lump: Full examination of lump

- Nodule: Look for "triggering effect"

- Cords: Passively extend fingers and palpate for possible cords in palm (Dupuytren's)

- Autonomous sensory areas:

    - <u>Tip of index finger:</u> Median nerve

    - <u>Base of thenar area:</u> Palmar cutaneous branch of median nerve

    - <u>Tip of little finger:</u> Ulnar nerve

    - <u>Dorsum of 5th metacarpal:</u> Dorsal cutaneous branch of ulnar nerve

    - <u>Dorsal 1st webspace:</u> Radial nerve

Move

Assess active and then passive ROM.

- Composite movement: Look for extension and flexion of fingers (fingertip to palm distance can be used as a quick measure of movement loss)
- Finger joints:
    - DIP: 0-80 degrees
    - PIP: 0-100 degrees
    - MCP: 0-40 degrees hyperextension to 90 degrees flexion
- Thumb:
    - Extension (sideways movement in the plane of the palm)
    - Abduction (upward movement at right angle to the palm)
    - Adduction (pressing against the palm)
    - Flexion (sideways movement across the palm)
    - Opposition (touching the tips of the fingers)
    - Retropulsion (lifting the thumb backwards behind the plane of the hand)

Muscles and Tendons

1. FDP: Immobilize PIP in extension and ask to flex DIP joint

2. FDS of non-index fingers: Grasp all fingers in extension (FDP with common belly is restricted), except the one being tested and ask to flex the isolated finger

3. FDS of index finger: Ask to pinch hard with DIP in extension and PIP in full flexion (FDP of index finger has a separate belly)

4. FPL: Immobilize thumb MCP in extension and ask to flex IP joint

5. EPL: Check retropulsion of thumb

6. Long extensors: Ask to extend MCP joint

7. EIP (found on ulnar side of EDC): Ask to flex MCP joints of all other fingers (defunction EDC), and extend index finger actively; can be used for tendon transfer

8. Intrinsic muscles: Ask to make 'duckbill' position, i.e. Flex MCP joints and extend IP joints simultaneously

9. PL (Schaeffer's test): Ask to oppose thumb to little finger and flex the wrist (useful for tendon transfers); absent in 15%

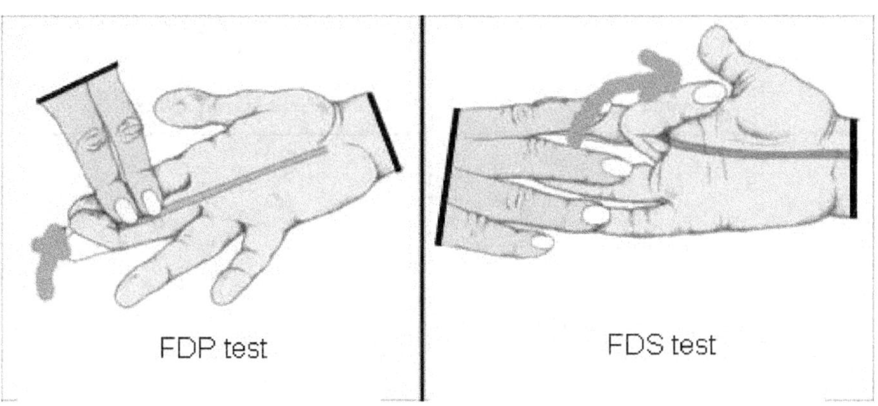

Grip

1. Pick a pin: Precision grip

2. Hold a sheet of paper: Pinch grip

3. Hold a pen: Tripod/chuck grip

4. Hold a key (side to end): Key grip

5. Hold my curled fingers: Hook group

6. Grip my forearm: Grasp/span

7. Handshake: Power grip

8. Grip strength: Ask patient to squeeze partially inflated sphygmomanometer cuff (20 mmHg) – normally a pressure of 150 mmHg can be achieved easily

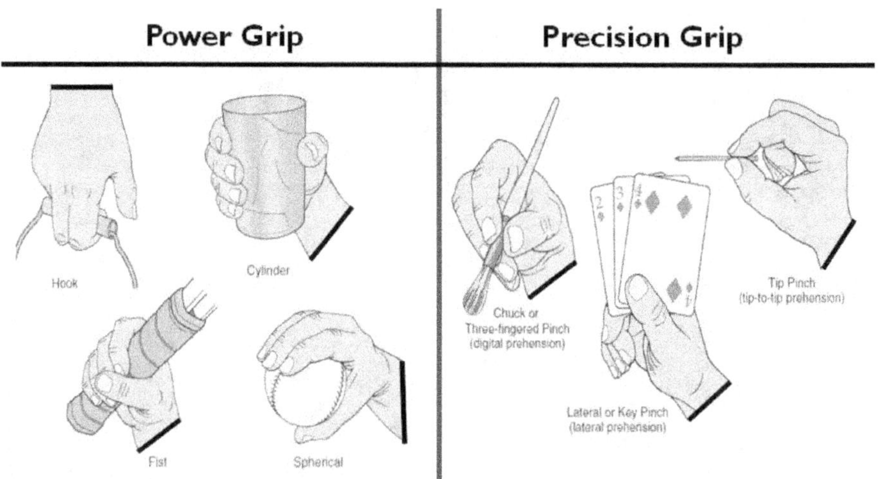

Special tests

1. **Allen's test:** Patient clenches fist several times before making a fist (exsanguination), then examiner occludes radial and ulnar artery simultaneously with fingers. Ask the patient to release fist (must stay blanched, else the occlusion pressure is not adequate). Release compressed arteries one at a time to test that artery. Normal color

must return within 5-15 seconds. **Digital Allen's test** is similar to Allen's test but digital arteries are occluded.

2. **Bunnel's test:** Assess passive PIP joint flexion in 2 positions:

- In MCP extension (intrinsics in tension) < In MCP flexion (intrinsics relaxed): Intrinsic tightness
- In MCP extension (extrinsics relaxed) > In MCP flexion (extrinsics tightened): Extrinsic tightness
- Limited in both MCP extension and flexion: Capsular tightness

3. **Bouvier's test:** In a claw hand, correct MCP hyperextension – if the patient is able to extend IP joints (tenodesis working), then the clawing is flexible.

4. **Elson test:** Ask to place the patient's hand flat on table with PIP joint flexed over the edge of table. Ask to actively extend finger against resistance:

- Intact central slip: Strong PIP extension (central slip works) and Relaxed DIP (lateral bands will remain slack due to tethering of extensor mechanism by central slip)

- <u>Ruptured central slip:</u> Weak PIP extension (central slip defunctions) and Hyperextension and stiffness of DIP (lateral band tensioning)

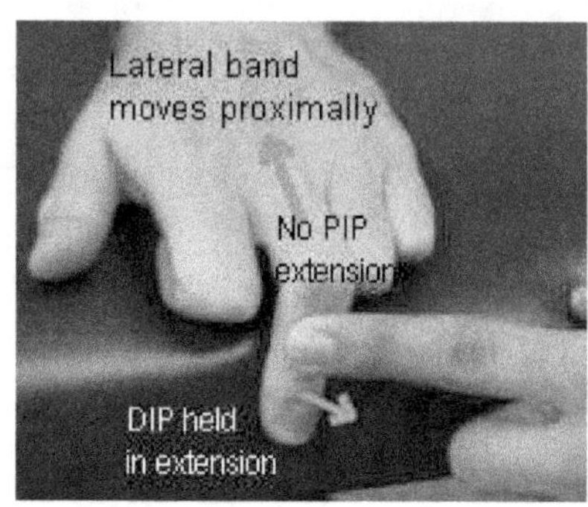

5. Test for ORL tightness: Assess passive flexion of DIP in 2 positions:

- <u>In PIP flexion (relaxes ORL) > In PIP extension:</u> ORL tightness
- <u>In PIP flexion = In PIP extension:</u> DIP contracture

6. 1st MCP valgus stress test:

- <u>Instability in neutral (0°):</u> Injury to proper and accessory UCL and/or volar plate
- <u>Instability in 30° flexion:</u> Injury to proper UCL

Examination of Peripheral Nerves - discussed separately here

CHAPTER 14

Foot & Ankle Examination

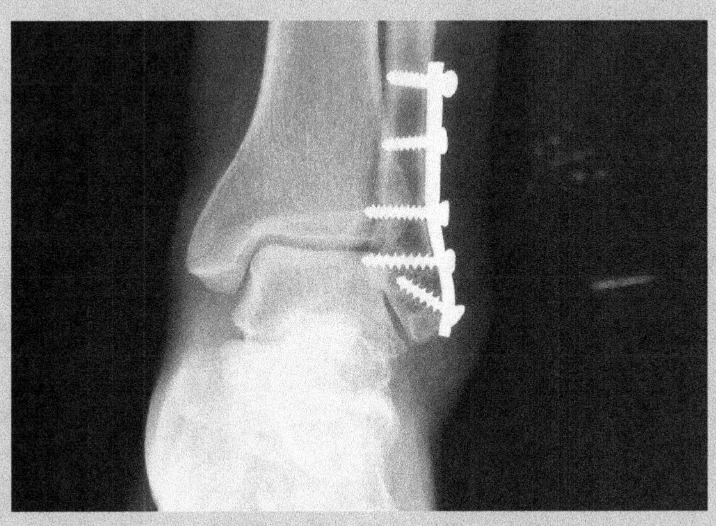

Foot and Ankle Examination

The clinical examination of foot and ankle must be done with the patient in both weight-bearing and non-weight bearing positions. It should proceed in a systematic manner as highlighted earlier including the examination of gait.

Look

Look for **SEADS GO**.

A. Standing

1. <u>From behind:</u>

- Asymmetry of calves

- Swelling of Achilles tendon or posteromedial or posterolateral aspect of ankle

- Tibiocalcaneal angle (usually 5 degrees valgus)

- Visible forefoot (normally 1 and 1/2 toes):

- "too many toes" sign (forefoot abduction in tibialis posterior dysfunction)
- Lumbar spine for signs of dysraphism

2. <u>From anterior:</u>

- Peek-a-boo sign (visualization of medial side of heel in cavo-varus)
- Ankle swelling (synovitis, effusion, osteophytes)
- Medial longitudinal arch (normal, planus, cavus)
- Midfoot deformities
- Forefoot deformities:
    - Start with hallux and go laterally
        - Lateral deviation of hallux: Hallux valgus
        - PIP flexion and MTP extension (like boutonniere): Hammer toe
        - DIP and PIP flexion and MTP extension (like intrinsic minus): Claw toe
        - DIP flexion (like mallet finger): Mallet toe
    - Skin and nail changes

2. Gait
([https://epomedicine.com/clinical-medicine/physical-exa](https://epomedicine.com/clinical-medicine/physical-examination-gait/))
mination-gait/))

3. Rise on tiptoes (heel raise): screens for functioning gastroc-soleus complex

- Heel adopts varus: Functioning tibialis posterior tendon

b. Sitting/Lying: Examine plantar aspect

- Keratoses
- Ulcer
- Orthosis, shoe wear, walking aids

Feel

Feel for **TEST Areas**:

Follow a systematic approach in a clockwise fashion from medial to anterior to lateral to posterior.

- Harty notch (space medial to tibialis anterior tendon): synovitis, effusion or crepitus can be felt here
- Feel pulses (D.pedis absent in 1/6 patients)
- If a neuropathy suspected, test vibration sense, protective sensation and sense of position
- Anterolateral impingement test:
  - Thumb pressure applied over the anterolateral gutter with the foot in plantarflexion will push any hypertrophic synovium into the joint causing pain. If the foot is then moved into dorsiflexion the pain intensifies which is positive for synovial impingement.
- Inferior tibiofibular syndesmosis:
  - Tenderness
  - Squeeze test: Squeeze at mid-calf level provokes pain
  - Dorsiflexion-eversion test: provokes pain
- Ankle ligaments:
  - Anterior drawer test (for ATFL):
    - Knee joint in flexion and ankle in 10-15 degrees plantar flexion

- Maneuver: The examiner exerts a downward force on the tibia while simultaneously attempting to "lift up" the foot while grasping behind the heel.
        - Interpretation: A significant difference from the unaffected side (>2 mm) or dimpling of the anterior skin (suction or dimple sign) is considered positive.
    - Talar tilt test:
        - Positioned in sitting or supine lying with the knee in full extension. Examiner stabilizes distal leg with one hand while the other hand holds the heel with ankle to assess:
        - ATFL : Plantar flexion – inversion
        - CFL: Neutral position – inversion
        - PTFL: Dorsiflexion – inversion
        - Deltoid ligament: Plantar flexion – eversion
- Sinus tarsi: tenderness in subtalar joint irritation
- Tendon thickening: moves with tendon movement

- Tendon sheath thickening: doesn't move with movement of tendon
- Tenderness of anteromedial tuberosity of calcaneus: Plantar fasciitis
- Side-to-side compression of calcaneus: Calcaneal fracture
- Windlass effect/Jack's test (Passively dorsiflex great toe): Tenses plantar fascia and recreates pain (plantar fasciitis) and restores medial longitudinal arch (flexible flat foot)
- 2nd metatarsal shaft tenderness: Stress fracture
- 2nd MTP joint swelling & tenderness: Freiberg's disease
- MTP synovitis:
  - 'Daylight' sign: synovitis pushes toes apart so daylight can be seen between each
  - 'Squeeze' test: discomfort
- Tenderness between metatarsal heads (esp. 3rd web space) with burning and paresthesia: Morton's neuroma
  - Mulder's click or sign: Squeeze and dorsal directed pressure from plantar aspect of webspace produces click

- Pain beneath MTP joint: Sesamoiditis, Degenerative process, AVN, stress fracture

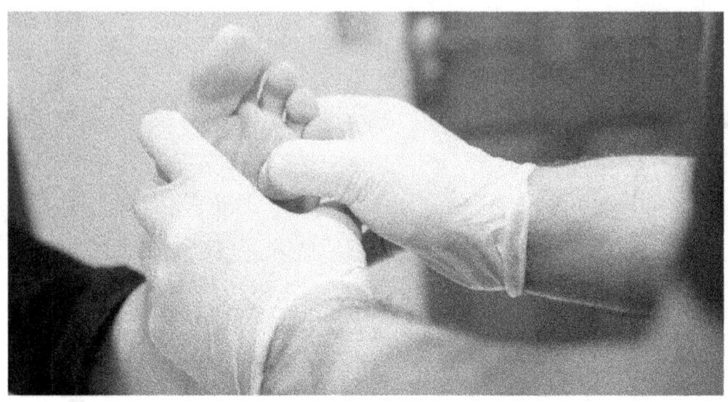

[File:Mulder's Click Test for Morton's Neuroma.jpg - WikiSM](#)

Move

Perform passive then the active ROM from 'neutral' position of foot.

a. **Ankle:** Passive movement must be assessed with forefoot in supination and inversion of heel (to exclude dorsiflexion at chopart's joint and midtarsal joint and to lock subtalar joint).

With legs hanging from couch (knee flexion) and knee extension:

- Dorsiflexion: 0-15 degrees

- Plantarflexion: 0-40 degrees

<u>Silfverskiold test for decreased ankle dorsiflexion:</u>

- Dorsiflexion in knee flexion> in knee extension: isolated gastrocnemius contracture

- Dorsiflexion in knee flexion = in knee extension: both gastrocnemius and soleus contracture

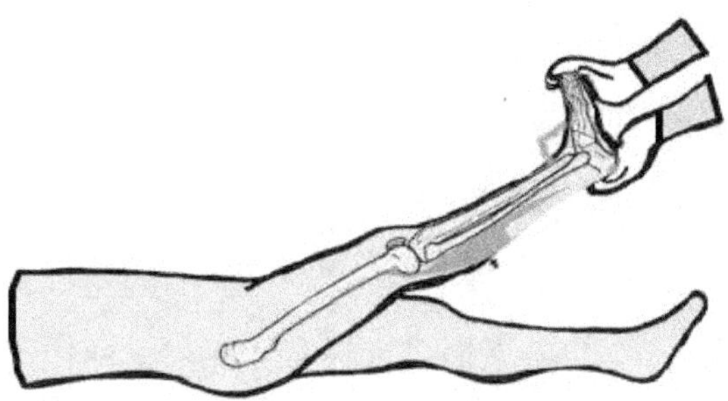

Ankle dorsiflexion in knee extension

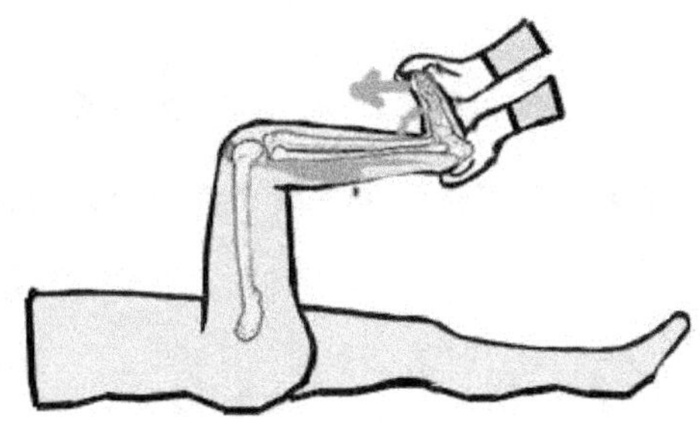

Ankle dorsiflexion in knee flexion

b. **Subtalar:** Lock ankle by ensuring plantigrade position when heel is moved –

- Inversion: 30 degrees
- Eversion: 15 degrees

c. **Midtarsal:** Fix calcaneus (heel) with 1 hand and move forefoot:

- Abduction: 5 degrees
- Adduction: 5 degrees

d. **Mobility of 1st TMT joint:** Fix tarsals with 1 hand and move 1st metatarsal up and down (may be contributing factor in hallux valgus and may need Lapidus fusion)

e. **Toes:**

- Dorsiflexion of great toe at MTP: 70 degrees
- Plantar flexion of great toe at MTP: 10 degrees

Neurovascular Examination

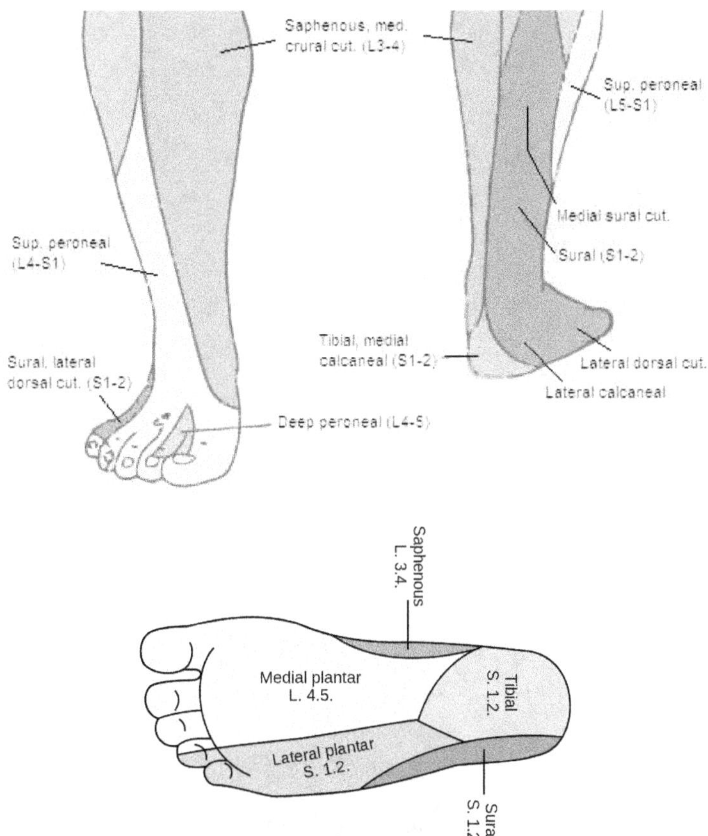

By Henry Vandyke Carter - Henry Gray (1918) Anatomy of the Human Body (See "Book" section below)Bartleby.com: Gray's Anatomy, Plate 826, Public Domain, https://commons.wikimedia.org/w/index.php?curid=3429653

- **Neurologic:** Motor, Sensory, Reflex (Achilles tendon reflex)
- **Vascular:** D. pedis, Tibialis posterior, CRT

Special tests

1. Coleman block test:

- Indication: Cavovarus foot to differentiate if it is fore-foot driven or hind-foot driven and if it is fixed or flexible
    - Fore-foot driven: Neuromuscular causes (CMT, spinal dysraphism)
        - Tripod effect (1st MT head, calcaneus, 3rd MT head): Plantar flexed 1st MT (due to sparing of peroneus longus) pulls hindfoot into varus
    - Hindfoot driven: Trauma (varus malunion of talus fractures)
- 2.5 cm (1 inch) block or book is placed under foot such that 1st ray is unsupported
    - Hindfoot varus corrects: Fore-foot driven and the hindfoot is flexible
    - Hindfoot varus doesn't correct: Hind-foot driven or hindfoot is rigid

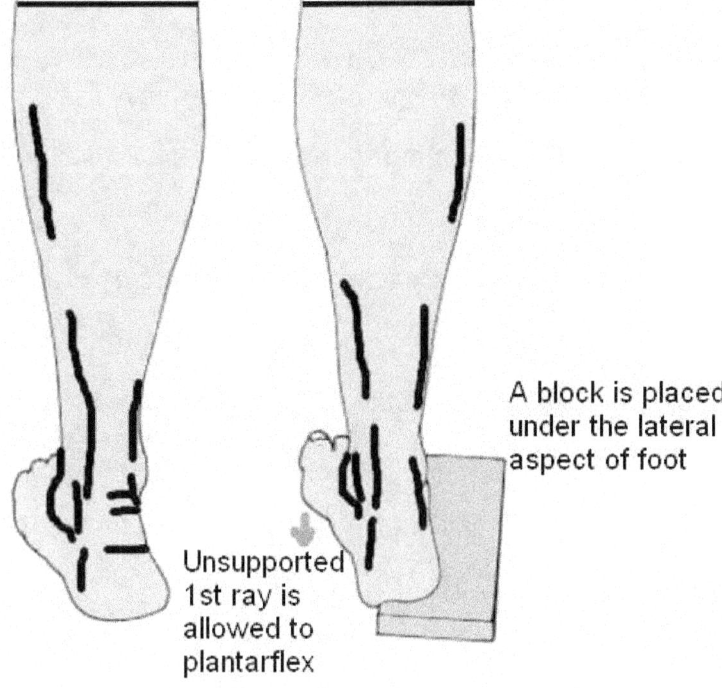

2. **Single leg tiptoe test (heel raise):**

- Near wall so that patient can lean to support

- Standing on tip-toe: normally heel will go into varus and medial longitudinal arch is elevated (windlass effect)

- If tibialis posterior tendon dysfunction:
    - Double heel raise: affected foot remains in valgus
    - Single heel raise: cannot perform on affected side

3. **Tests for achilles tendon integrity:**

- <u>Simmond-Thompson test:</u> Patient kneels or lies prone with feet hanging of the table, & the examiner squeezes the calf:
  - Normal (Intact): Produces plantar flexion
  - Positive (Rupture): No plantar flexion
- <u>Matle's test:</u> Patient lies prone with knee flexed perpendicular and foot/ankle in neutral
  - Positive: More dorsiflexed ankle on the side of rupture

4. **Muscles around ankle:**

- Tibialis posterior: Resisted inversion at plantarflexion
- Tibialis anterior: Resisted dorsiflexion with some inversion
- Peroneus longus: Resisted plantarflexion and eversion
- Peroneus brevis: Resisted eversion in neutral position

CHAPTER 15

Median Nerve Examination

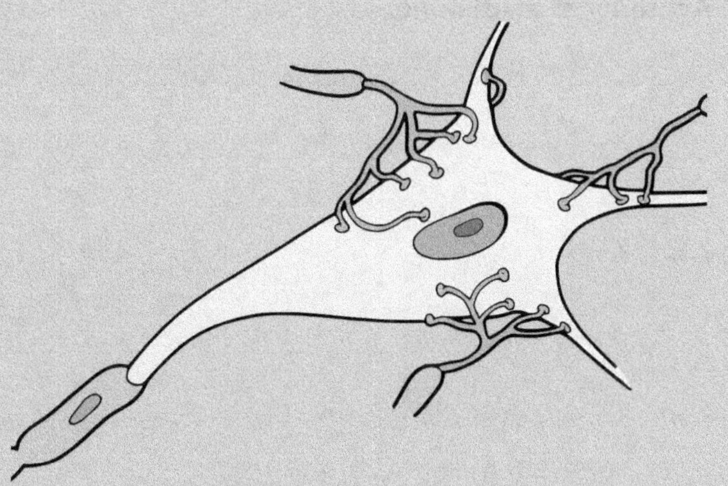

Median Nerve Examination

The median nerve predominantly provides motor innervation to the flexor muscles of the forearm and hand. The median nerve also provides sensory innervation to the dorsal aspect (nail bed) of the distal first two digits of the hand, the palmar aspect of the thumb, index, middle, and half of the ring finger, the palm, as well as the medial aspect of the forearm.

Anatomy of median nerve:

https://epomedicine.com/medical-students/median-ulnar-and-radial-nerve-course-and-innervation/

Look

1.	Wasting of thenar muscles particularly APB

2.	Wasting for forearm muscles

3.	**Ape or Simian hand deformity:** Due to inefficiency of the APB and OP, the 1st metacarpal drops to the same plane as the other metacarpals.

4.   Relevant scars

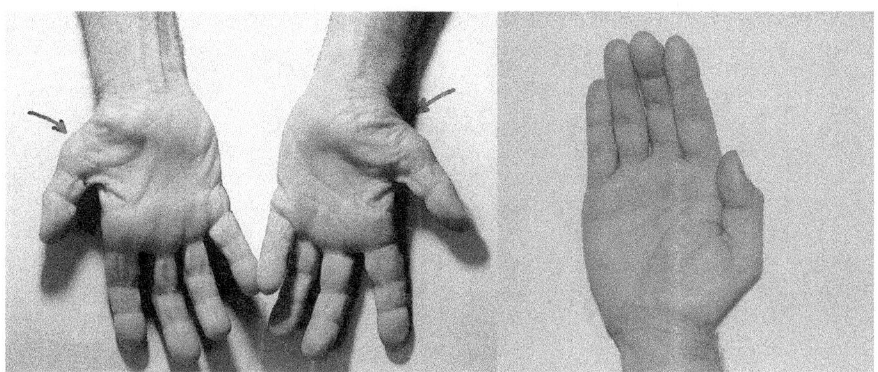

Left: Thenar wasting (Dr. Harry Gouvas, MD, PhD, Public domain,

via Wikimedia Commons)

Right: Simian hand (Emily Barrett, CC BY 3.0, via Wikimedia Commons)

Screen

Pointing index sign (Benedict sign) – In high median nerve palsy due to affection of FDS and FDP to the index finger, the index finger cannot be flexed. The other fingers can due to the action of the ulnar half of FDP supplied by the ulnar nerve.

OK sign – Instruct the patient to make an "O" with index finger & thumb. The patient cannot make an "O" without hyperextending the IPJ in cases of AIN palsy.

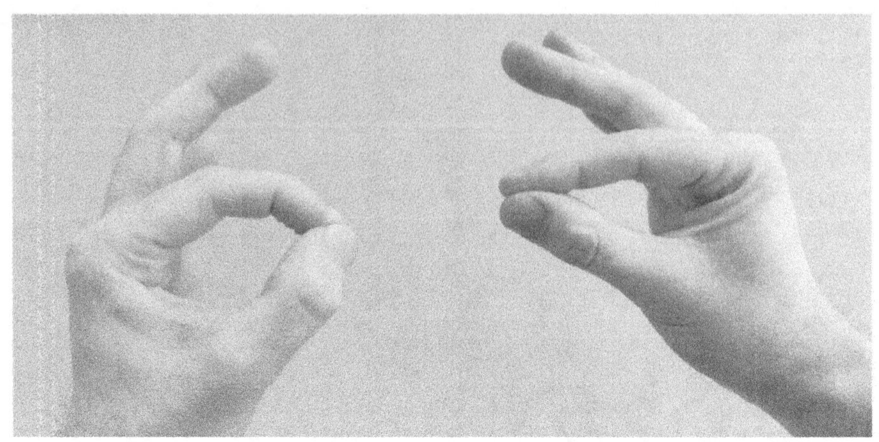

Left – normal; Right – AIN injury

Löppönen P, Hulkkonen S, Ryhänen J. Proximal Median Nerve Compression in the Differential Diagnosis of Carpal Tunnel Syndrome. *Journal of Clinical Medicine.* 2022; 11(14):3988. https://doi.org/10.3390/jcm11143988 [CC-BY 4.0]

Feel

a. Sensation:

- <u>At tip of index finger:</u> Tests median nerve terminal branch
- <u>At thenar eminence:</u>
    - Loss of sensation: Injury proximal to carpal tunnel (palmar cutaneous branch arises 3-5 cm proximal to wrist crease and travels

superficial to the transverse carpal

ligament)

b. Palpation:

- ○ <u>Tenderness:</u> Over the course of median nerve in proximal forearm at the sites of compression

Move (Motor testing)

a. Muscles supplied proximal to carpal tunnel:

- <u>FCR:</u> Instruct the patient to flex the wrist against resistance while palpating the FCR tendon
- <u>FDS:</u> Ask the patient to place hand flat on the table with palms facing upwards. Hold the fingers (except the one to be tested) in extension and instruct the patient to bend the finger to be tested and observe for active flexion at the PIP joint.

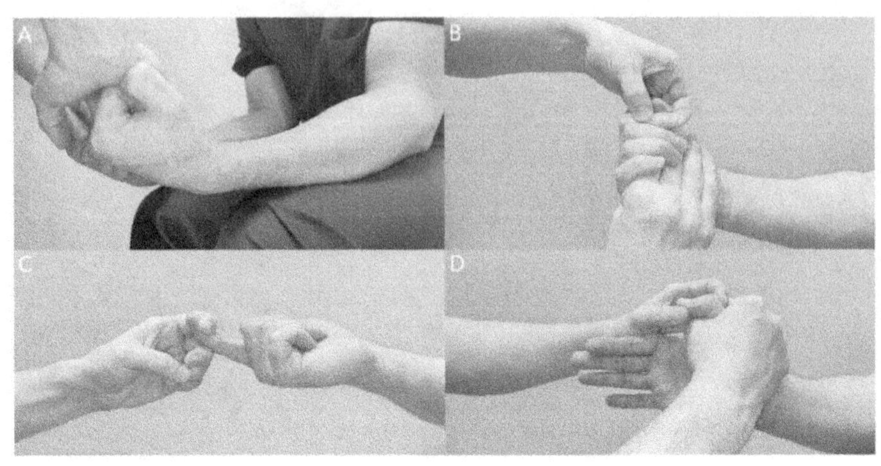

A – FCR; B & C – FDP; D – FPL

Löppönen P, Hulkkonen S, Ryhänen J. Proximal Median Nerve Compression in the Differential Diagnosis of Carpal Tunnel Syndrome. *Journal of Clinical Medicine.* 2022; 11(14):3988. https://doi.org/10.3390/jcm11143988 [CC-BY 4.0]

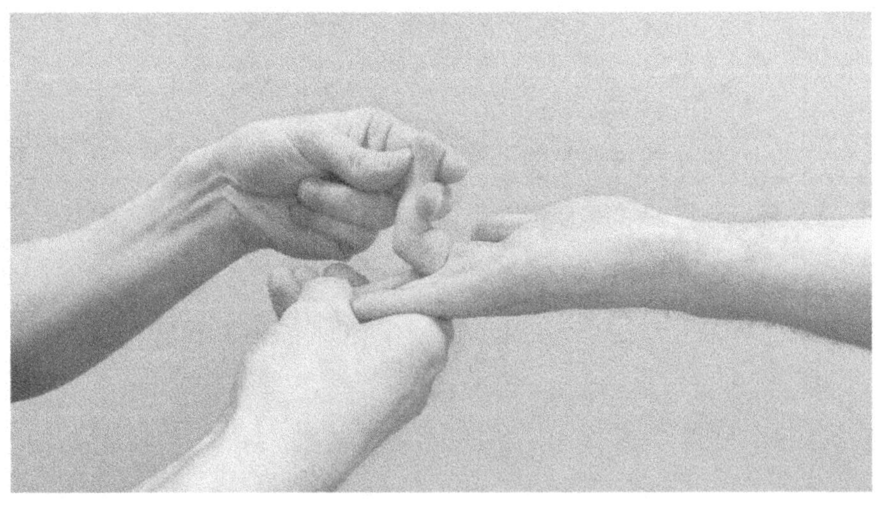

FDS test

Löppönen P, Hulkkonen S, Ryhänen J. Proximal Median Nerve Compression in the Differential Diagnosis of Carpal Tunnel Syndrome. *Journal of Clinical Medicine*. 2022; 11(14):3988. https://doi.org/10.3390/jcm11143988 [CC-BY 4.0]

b. Muscles supplied distal to carpal tunnel:

- <u>APB:</u> Ask the patient to place hand flat on the table with palms facing upwards. Instruct the patient to raise the thumb towards the ceiling against resistance or touch the pen held above the thumb (pen test) while palpating the APB muscles (most lateral of the thenar muscle)
- <u>OP:</u> Ask the patient to touch the tip of thumb to the tip of little finger firmly while resisting the pull by examiner

c. AIN: Ask the patient to make "O" with the tip of thumb and tip of index finger (Bunnell's OK sign) –

- <u>AIN intact (FPL & FDP):</u> Patient can make "O"
- <u>AIN injured:</u> Patient hyperextends the IPJ of thumb and DIPJ of index finger in an attempt to make an "O"

Provocation tests

a. **Pronator syndrome:** Reproduction of symptoms by –

1. <u>Resisted elbow flexion with forearm supinated</u> or <u>Resisted supination with elbow flexed</u> (bicipital aponeurosis/lacertus fibrosus)
2. <u>Resisted forearm pronation with elbow extended</u> (at 2 heads of pronator teres)
3. <u>Resisted PIPJ flexion of middle finger</u> (FDS fibrous arch)
4. Positive <u>Tinel sign in the proximal anterior forearm</u> but no Tinel sign at wrist

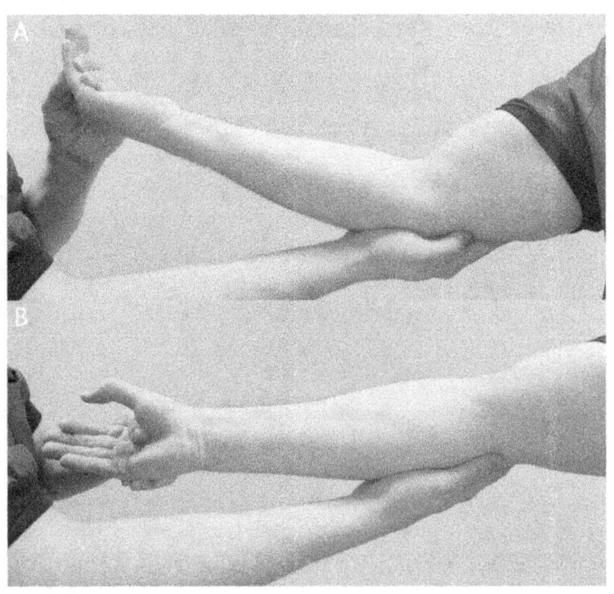

Lacertus fibrosus entrapment test

Löppönen P, Hulkkonen S, Ryhänen J. Proximal Median Nerve Compression in the Differential Diagnosis of Carpal Tunnel Syndrome. *Journal of Clinical Medicine.* 2022; 11(14):3988. https://doi.org/10.3390/jcm11143988 [CC-BY 4.0]

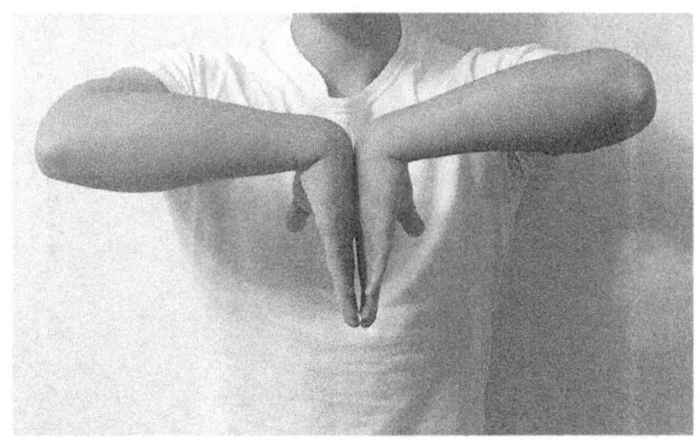

Phalen's test

LittleT889, CC BY-SA 4.0, via Wikimedia Commons

b. **Carpal tunnel syndrome:** Reproduction of symptoms by –

1. <u>Phalen's test:</u> Maximally flexing wrist reproduces symptoms within 60 seconds
   a. Time dependent: Shorter the time taken, more sensitive the test
2. <u>Reverse Phalen's test:</u> Placing the wrist in position of maximum extension
3. <u>Carpal tunnel compression (Durkan) test:</u> Direct pressure applied with both thumbs over the carpal tunnel (forearm supinated & wrist in neutral) reproduces symptoms within 30 seconds
4. <u>Wrist flexion and carpal tunnel compression test:</u> Combination of Phalen's test and Durkan test
   a. Reproduces symptoms within 20 seconds
5. <u>Tourniquet test & Straight arm raising test:</u> Nerve ischemia generated by either applying a tourniquet or elevating the arm above the head level with wrist in neutral position
6. <u>Tinel's test:</u> Percussion of the median nerve just proximal to the wrist crease at the point at which the nerve enters the carpal tunnel reproduces symptoms

CHAPTER 16

Ulnar Nerve Examination

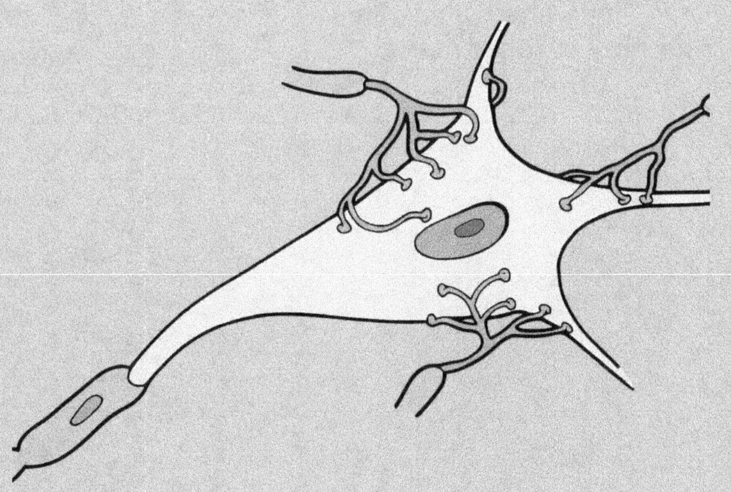

Ulnar Nerve Examination

The ulnar nerve arises from the medial cord of the brachial plexus. It contains the nerve root fibers from C8 to T1. It provides the motor supply to the hypothenar muscles, the ulnar 2 lumbricals, the interosseous muscles, the adductor pollicis, FCU, and the FDP to the ring and small fingers. Its sensory distribution includes the palmar surface of the small and the ulnar half of the ring finger as well as the dorsoulnar carpus.

Anatomy of ulnar nerve:

https://epomedicine.com/medical-students/ulnar-nerve-cour se-and-innervation/

Look

- **Rectangle palm sign:** Normal square shape palm becomes rectangular with severe wasting of hypothenar eminence & 1st dorsal interosseous muscle

- **Masse sign:** Wasting of hypothenar eminence and flattened palmar metacarpal arch
- **Wasting of volar ulnar side of forearm (FCU & FDP):** With proximal injury of nerve
- Relevant scars
- **Wartenberg's sign (Little finger escape):** Little finger adopts abducted posture (weakness of ulnar nerve innervated 3rd palmar interosseous muscle + overpowering by PIN innervated EDM)
- **Clawing or Duchenne's sign or Hand of Benediction (at rest):** Hyperextension at MCPJ & Flexion at PIPJ (opposite of lumbrical function)
  - Index and middle finger are less affected (supplied by median nerve)
  - Ulnar paradox (clawing appears more severe with distal ulnar nerve lesions as FDP to ring and little finger which is responsible for DIPJ flexion is spared)
    - With high ulnar nerve injury – clawing initially worsens as the nerve recovers and begins to reinnervate FDP

- ○ <u>Bouvier's maneuver/sign</u> (dorsal pressure or downward force over the proximal phalanges corrects most of the clawing because EDC can extend PIPJ and DIPJ after prevention of MCPJ hyperextension)
  - ○ <u>Andre-Thomas sign</u> (clawing is made worse by an unconscious effort to extend the fingers by tenodesing the extensor tendons with palmar flexion of wrist)

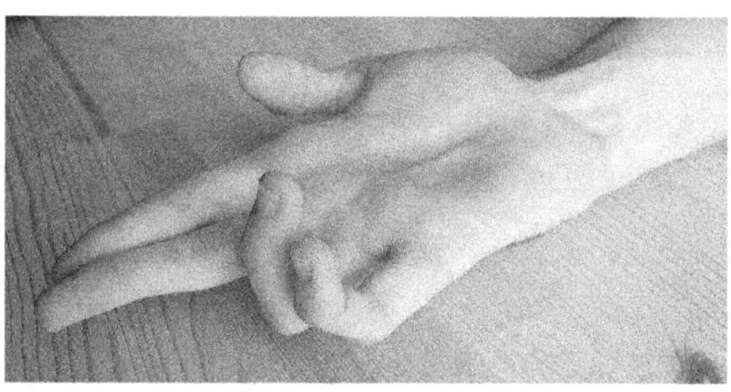

Ulnar claw hand

Mcstrother, CC BY 3.0, via Wikimedia Commons

Screen

Crossed finger test: Instruct the patients to cross fingers – if the patient cannot, it denotes interosseous muscle dysfunction.

Instruct the patient to make a fist – if the patient cannot tuck in little finger & ring finger, it denotes dysfunction of FDP to 4th & 5th finger.

Feel

a. **Sensation:**

- Sensory loss over dorsum of 5th metacarpal + Sensory loss over tip of little finger = Proximal pathology (like at Cubital tunnel)
- Sensation intact over dorsum of 5th metacarpal + Sensory loss over tip of little finger = Low lesion (Guyon's canal)

b. **Palpation:**

- Tenderness at:
    - Cubital tunnel (differentiate from medial epicondylitis)
    - Guyon's canal

Move (Motor testing)

a. Forearm muscles:

- <u>FCU (Flexor carpi ulnaris):</u> Resisted wrist flexion while palpating the FCU tendon to feel tension
- <u>FDP (Flexor digitorum profundus):</u> Resisted DIPJ flexion of little finger while the examiner stabilizes PIPJ
  - Inability to flex DIPJ of little and ring finger = Pollock's sign

b. Hand muscles:

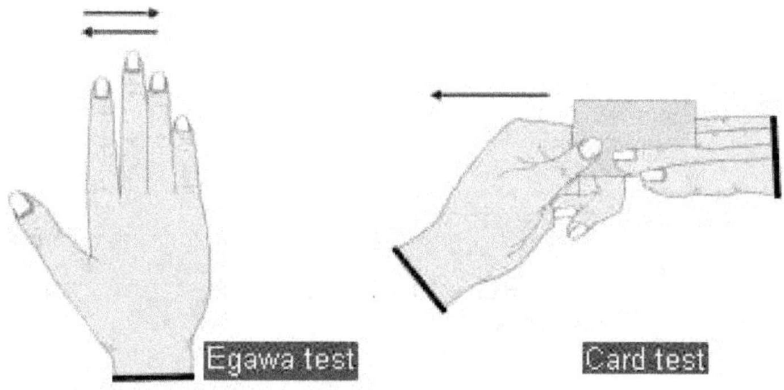

- <u>ADM (Abductor digiti minimi):</u> Resisted abduction of little finger with forearm in supination & wrist in neutral

- <u>Interossei muscles:</u>
  - Dorsal interossei (dAb = Abduction):
    - <u>Egawa's test:</u> Place the hand flat on table and ask the patient to move middle finger sideways
    - <u>Pitres-Testut sign:</u> Place the hand flat on table and ask the patient to move extended middle finger sideways
    - <u>Resisted abduction of index finger</u> while the examiner holds the hand and palpates the muscle to feel for tension
    - Palmar interossei (pAd = Adduction):
      - <u>Card test:</u> A card is inserted between 2 extended fingers & the patient is asked to grasp it between the fingers while the clinician gently tries to pull the card

- <u>AdPB (Adductor Pollicis Brevis):</u>
  - ○ Froment's sign or Book test: Ask the patient to hold a piece of paper or a book between their thumb & index finger
    - ■ Ulnar nerve palsy: Compensatory thumb IPJ flexion (recruitment of AIN innervated FPL) + Hyper-extension of MCPJ of thumb (Jeanne's sign)
    - ■ Normal: Patient can hold the card/book with adduction of thumb

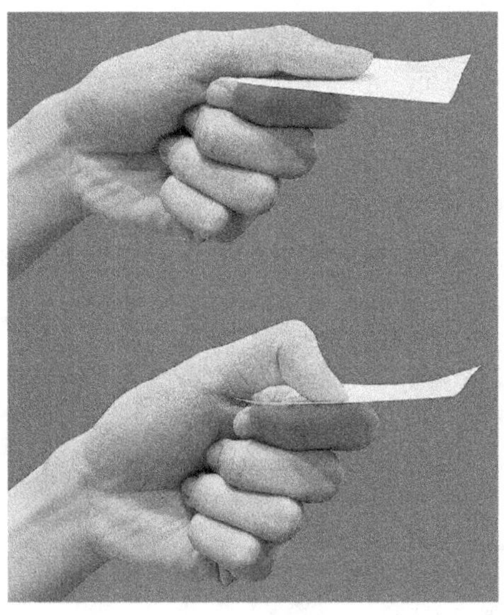

Froment's sign
Athikhun.suw, CC BY-SA 4.0, via Wikimedia Commons

Provocation tests

a. Cubital tunnel syndrome:

1. <u>Elbow flexion test:</u> Maximum flexion of elbow with extension of wrist & fingers for >60 seconds reproduces symptoms

2. <u>Pressure provocation test:</u> Pressure applied to ulnar nerve by middle and index finger immediately proximal to cubital tunnel for 60 seconds reproduces symptoms

3. <u>Tinel's sign:</u> Percussion of ulnar nerve over cubital tunnel

b. Guyon's canal:

1. <u>Tinel's sign:</u> Percussion of ulnar nerve over guyon's canal

2. <u>Allen Test:</u> Evaluates the arterial supply of the hand, which is useful when Ulnar Artery Thrombosis is suspected.

CHAPTER 17

Radial Nerve Examination

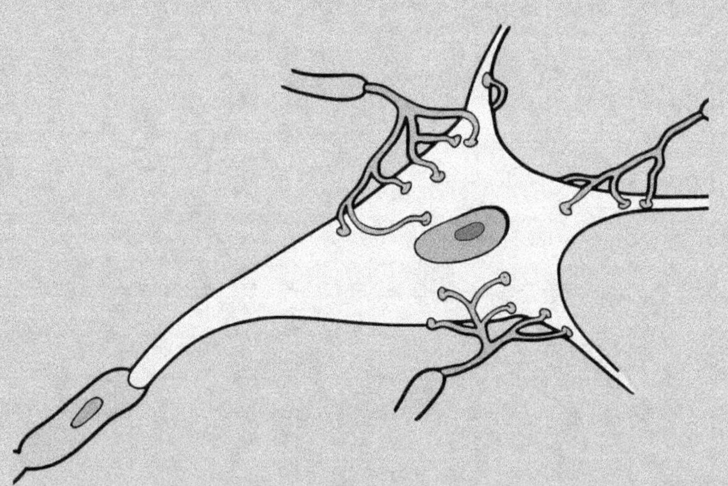

Radial Nerve Examination

The radial nerve stems from the posterior cord of the brachial plexus and supplies the upper limb. It also supplies the triceps brachii muscle of the arm, the muscles in the posterior compartment of the forearm (also known as the extensors), the wrist joint capsule, and aspects of the dorsal skin of the forearm and hand.

Anatomy of radial nerve:

https://epomedicine.com/clinical-medicine/examination-of-radial-nerve-palsy-or-injury/

Look

1. Posture of wrist:
    a. Wrist and fingers drop
2. Use of wrist extension splint
3. Relevant scars

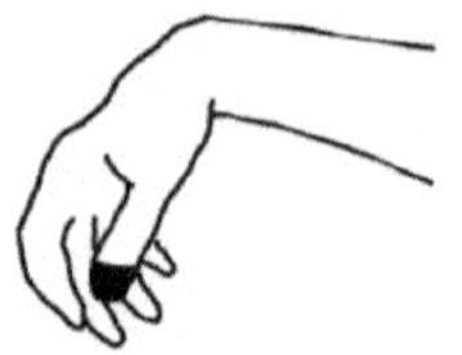

Central wrist drop
Clenching the fist leads to a
slight elevation of the hand.
Synkinetic wrist extension
intact.

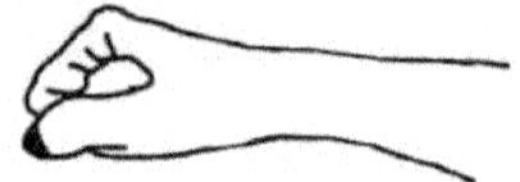

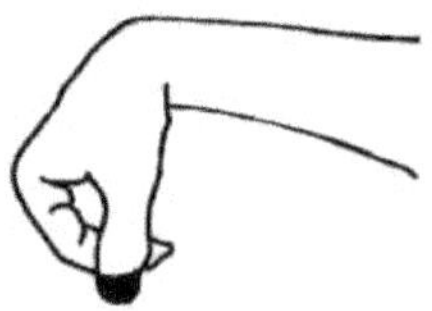

Peripheral wrist drop
clenching the fist leads to
worsening of the wrist drop.
Synkinetic wrist extension
impaired.

Rissardo JP, Byroju VV, Mukkamalla S, Caprara ALF. A Narrative Review of Stroke of Cortical Hand Knob Area. Medicina. 2024; 60(2):318. https://doi.org/10.3390/medicina60020318 [CC-BY 4.0]

Screen

Extension of index finger – Instruct the patient to point the finger.

Feel

a. **Sensation:** In the 1st webspace on hand dorsum

- Sensory loss:
    - Radial nerve palsy above bifurcation
    - Superficial sensory branch injury
- Weakness of muscle without sensory loss:
    - Posterior interosseous nerve (PIN) injury

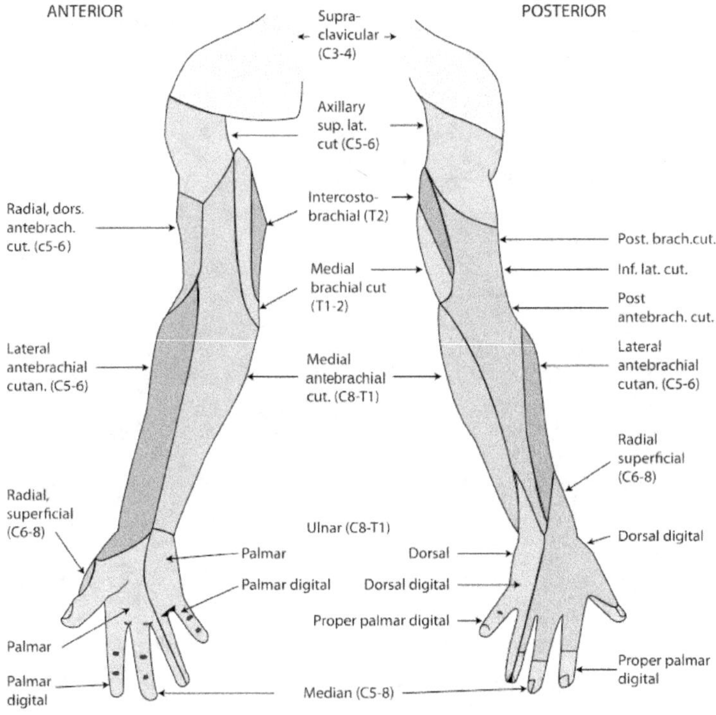

Henry Vandyke Carter, Public domain, via Wikimedia Commons

	Lateral epicondylitis	**Radial tunnel syndrome**
Tenderness	Lateral epicondyle	3-5 cm below lateral epicondyle on mobile wad

	Wartenberg's disease or Cheiralgia paresthetica	**De Quervain's syndrome**
Tenderness	Distally over superficial radial nerve	Radial styloid region
Tinel's sign	Positive	Negative

Move (Motor testing)

To test the muscles, the patient is asked to perform the particular muscle function against resistance and examiner palpates for the muscle. Examine the muscles in order of innervation.

Triceps: Eliminate gravity by placing the upper arm parallel to ground. Supporting the limb, ask the patient to

further extend the elbow against resistance from
half-extended position.

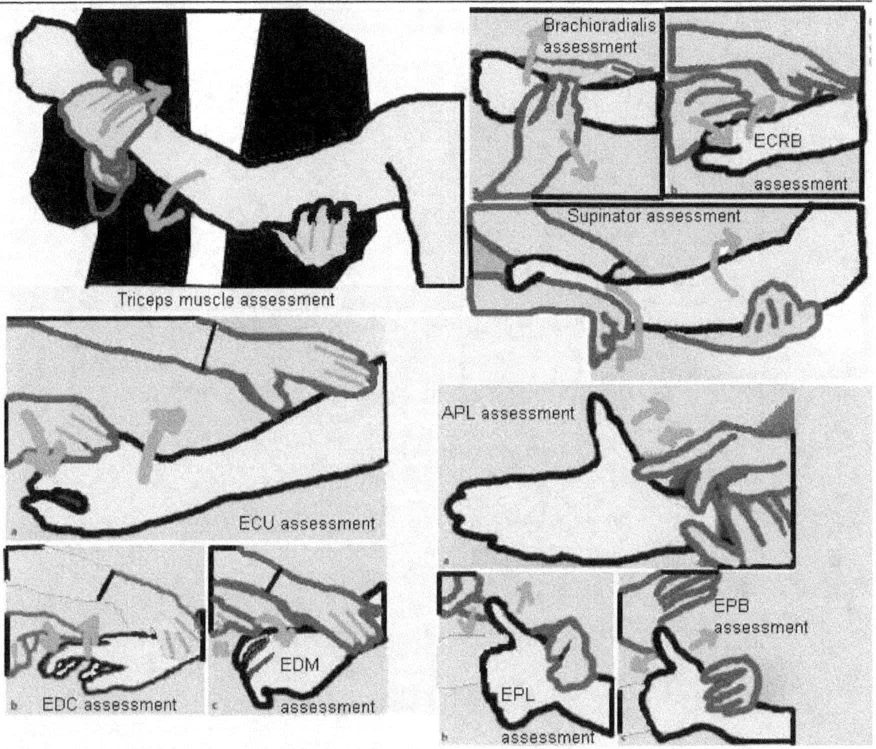

Lateral epicondyle group:

1. <u>Brachioradialis:</u> As the patient flexes forearm against resistance in neutral position, brachioradialis is felt in lateral antecubital fossa.

2. <u>ECRL and ECRB:</u> Ask the patient to extend and adduct the wrist against resistance with the forearm pronated and feel the muscle.

3. <u>Supinator:</u> With the forearm extended (to minimize the role of biceps), the patient is asked to resist pronation and muscle is felt.

PIN – superficial group:

1. <u>ECU:</u> Patient is asked to extend wrist in ulnar direction against resistance
2. <u>EDC:</u> With forearm in neutral position, patient is asked to extend MCP joint with resistance placed just proximal to PIP joint
   a. Extension of MCP joint is important because extension of IP joints with MCP in flexion is a function of intrinsic muscles supplied by the median and ulnar nerve.
3. <u>EDM:</u> Similar to EDC, but in little finger

PIN – deep group:

1. <u>APL:</u> Stabilize hand and ask the patient to extend MCP joint of thumb in radial direction against resistance (i.e. plane of palm).

2. <u>EPL:</u> With hand fisted, patient is asked to extend thumb against resistance placed over distal phalanx

3. <u>EPB:</u> With hand fisted, patient is asked to extend the thumb against resistance placed over proximal phalanx

Note: Abductor pollicis brevis (thenar muscle supplied by median nerve) abducts the thumb in a direction perpendicular to the plane of palm, i.e. towards the ceiling on a hand laid flat on floor.

Rex sign: In proximal third extensor aspect cut wound of forearm there can be inability to straighten the fingers or thumb that may be due to posterior interosseous nerve cut injury or muscle laceration. As abductor pollicis longus and extensor indicis has more distal origin in the forearm, if these muscles are functioning it indicates muscle laceration rather than posterior interosseous nerve injury at that level.

Provocation tests

a. Deep radial nerve (PIN) entrapment:

1. Proximal wrist pain with resisted wrist extension.

2. Extend elbow and pronate arm – resisted supination will lead to RTS symptoms.

3. Resisted middle finger extension compresses the PIN against the edge of ECRB, causing pain.

b. Superficial radial nerve entrapment: Forced forearm pronation reproduces symptoms within 1 minute (due to scissoring effect of ECRL and BR).

To differentiate high radial nerve palsy from a posterior interosseous nerve (PIN) palsy –

- High radial nerve palsy = Loss of all motor function + Loss of sensation in 1st webspace dorsum

- PIN palsy = Preserved brachioradialis and ECRL motor function + Spared sensation in 1st webspace dorsum

CHAPTER 18

Constructing Differentials

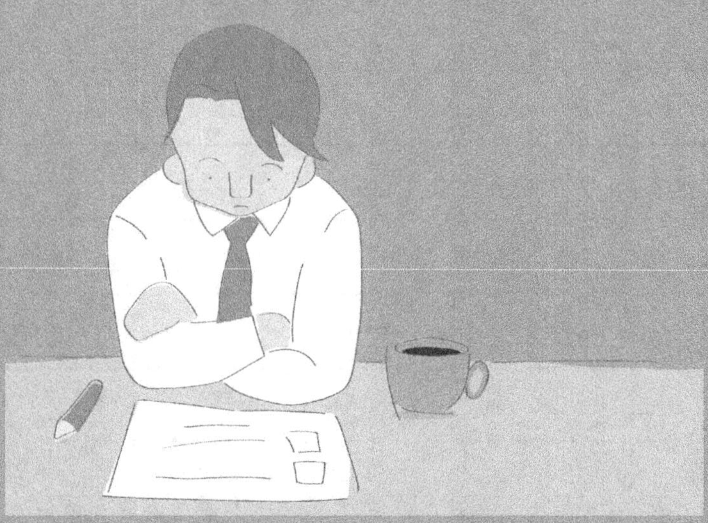

Constructing Differentials

Etiologic approach	Anatomic approach
<u>Mnemonic:</u> CHOPPED MINTS	<u>Intra-articular:</u>
1. Congenital	• Bone
2. Hematologic/Vascular	• Cartilage
3. Overuse	• Joint capsule
4. Psychogenic	• Synovium
5. Pregnancy-related	<u>Periarticular:</u>
6. Environmental	• Bursa
7. Degenerative	• Epiphysis/Apophysis
8. Metabolic or endocrine	• Tendon
9. Infectious/Inflammatory	• Bone
10. Neoplastic	• Skin/Fascia
11. Traumatic	• Muscle
12. Surgery-related	

Red Flag Signs: Indicate Non-mechanical pathology and may require immediate attention

History	Possible conditions
Constant & severe pain, esp. at night	Neoplasm, Acute injury
Unexplained wt. loss, Appetite loss	Neoplasm
Unusual fatigue	Neoplasm, Thyroid disorder
Frequent headaches, Visual blurring	Neoplasm
Arm pain lasting >2-3 months	Neoplasm, Neurologic
Persistent root pain	Neoplasm, Neurologic
Radicular pain with coughing	Neoplasm, Neurologic
Pain worsening after 1 month	Neoplasm
Paralysis, Paresthesia	Neoplasm, Neurologic
B/L nerve root signs & symptoms	Neoplasm, Spinal cord compression, VBI
Signs worse than symptoms	Neoplasm
Difficulty with balance & coordination	Spinal cord or CNS lesions
Fever or Night sweats	Systemic infections
Quadrilateral paresthesia	Cervical myelopathy, VBI

VBI: Vertebro-basilar Ischemia

Yellow Flag Signs: Potential confounding variables that may be cautionary warnings regarding the patient's condition & that require further investigation

Malingering: Intentional production of false symptoms or the exaggeration of symptoms that truly exist

Approach to joint pain:

https://epomedicine.com/clinical-medicine/mnemonic-based-approach-to-joint-pain/

Approach to low back pain:

https://epomedicine.com/medical-students/low-back-pain-lbp-made-easy/

Approach to heel pain:

https://epomedicine.com/clinical-medicine/heel-pain-mnemonic/

Index

www.ingramcontent.com/pod-product-compliance
Lightning Source LLC
Chambersburg PA
CBHW071452140726
47997CB00005B/1690